Dr Anita Mitra is an NHS doctor based in London specialising in gynaecology and gynaecological oncology, with experience in both clinical medicine and research. She is known as the Gynae Geek on social media, and this is also the title of her first book, published in 2019.

Also by Dr Anita Mitra:

The Gynae Geek: Your no-nonsense guide to 'down there' healthcare

Dealing with Problem Periods

DR ANITA MITRA

The information in this book may not be suitable for everyone and is not intended to be a substitute for medical advice or medical treatment. You are advised to consult a doctor on any matters relating to your health, and in particular on any matters that may require diagnosis or medical attention. Any use of the information in this book is made on the reader's good judgement after consulting with his or her doctor and is the reader's sole responsibility.

First published in paperback in 2024 by Headline Home
an imprint of Headline Publishing Group

1

Cataloguing in Publication Data is available from the British Library

Paperback ISBN 978 1035 40774 3
e-ISBN 978 1035 40775 0

Copy editor: Jane Hammett
Proofreader: Jill Cole
Indexer: Ruth Ellis
Typeset in Dante by CC Book Production
Printed and bound in Great Britain by Clays Ltd, Elcograf S.p.A.

MIX
Paper | Supporting responsible forestry
FSC® C104740
www.fsc.org

Headline's policy is to use papers that are natural, renewable and recyclable products and made from wood grown in well-managed forests and other controlled sources. The logging and manufacturing processes are expected to conform to the environmental regulations of the country of origin.

HEADLINE PUBLISHING GROUP
An Hachette UK Company
Carmelite House
50 Victoria Embankment
London
EC4Y 0DZ

www.headline.co.uk
www.hachette.co.uk

For my dad.

For inspiring me and providing me with the education that has allowed me to inspire and educate others.

Before we begin, I would like to touch on the language used throughout my book. You will see that I often use the words 'woman' and 'women' to refer to cis-gendered women with natal female anatomy. I strongly believe that healthcare should be inclusive, and I acknowledge that the words 'woman' and 'women' may not feel inclusive to everyone. In my clinical practice, I always strive to provide care that is compassionate, non-judgemental and personalised to each patient. To provide such personalisation in a book written for the general population is impossible to achieve but I hope the information discussed throughout might prompt anyone struggling with problem periods to try to access the individualised care that they deserve.

Contents

Introduction

This is a book about periods. It's for anyone who is experiencing problem periods, anyone who is supporting someone who has problem periods, or anyone who wants to learn more about periods: what they are, what they're supposed to be like, and what you can do when things go wrong.

I'm a gynaecologist, and every day in my working life I talk about periods. The same can be said for my non-working life too, because I'm often contacted by friends, and friends of friends, who have period-related questions and concerns. Many years ago, I felt a slight embarrassment when I was discussing periods, so trust me when I say I know that it can be awkward to talk about periods and our menstrual cycle.

But it's really important to normalise the conversation around periods, because doing this will help us to learn a lot about what's normal and what's not, and it can also make conversations with healthcare professionals that little bit easier.

I understand that women may feel that there are barriers to seeking medical advice, but it breaks my heart to hear that the reason someone has suffered with a health problem for so long is that they were too embarrassed or ashamed to tell someone about it. I have seen countless women over the years who felt they should not complain about problems relating to their periods, so I want to make it very clear that you should not feel afraid, guilty, or like you're wasting anyone's time if you're concerned about anything. As I always say, 'if it bothers you, bother someone about it'.

In the developed world, the average woman has 400 periods in her lifetime, which is ten times the number we had about one hundred years ago, when the average was about 40, due to the high number of pregnancies and subsequent breast-feeding-induced temporary cessation of periods (called lactational amenorrhoea – 'amenorrhoea' means that you don't have a menstrual cycle).[1] It's not surprising, therefore, that today periods are becoming increasingly problematic and have the potential to have a significant negative impact on quality of life.

I work in a very busy central London hospital, and all the information provided here is based on the current practice that you can expect from the NHS in England. It is referenced and based on current guidelines, as well as on my own opinions and my decade of experience working in gynaecology. I've quoted some figures to give you an idea of how common some problems, situations or risks may be, and for these I've provided references to scientific studies, but please be aware that your own doctor may quote a different figure based on their own experience and your personal situation.

You may notice that I frequently use the phrase 'it may' or 'there is a chance', and this is because very few things in life are certain, and the human body is not a textbook. I mention some medications, and the odd brand here and there, but I want to say here that I have no financial conflict of interest to declare. I've never been paid by a drug company to promote a drug – although for full disclosure, I once received a free pen from the company that makes Mirena®. . . I wrote this book to educate and empower women, with the ultimate goal of improving gynae health outcomes.

I hope you'll find this book educational, enlightening and supportive. Maybe it will give you the push you need to seek medical advice about something that has been bothering you for a while.

I'd love it if you could share this book with your friends, family, colleagues and support network, because sharing information about our health is one of the simplest ways in which we can start to improve our quality of life. We only have one life, and I want you to live yours to the full.

The first chapter begins by discussing the correct terminology to use for parts of our bodies, before going on to discuss all the issues that can be caused by periods.

Chapter 1

How our menstrual cycle works

I don't want this book to feel like a high-school biology lesson, but I think it's important to cover the basics. I've heard all the nicknames and pseudonyms you can think of for gynae anatomy during consultations at work, and at times this can make it difficult to understand where precisely my patient is referring to. On many occasions I've sought clarification: 'Do you mean your vagina?', which has been met with a sigh of relief, indicating that my patient realises this is a safe word to use, and invariably we can go on to have a clearer conversation, helping me to get to the bottom of things much faster and more concisely. The word 'vagina' is often used incorrectly to refer to the entire external genitalia. But did you know that your vag-IN-a is on the IN-side, and your vulva is the part on the outside?

Ultimately, I want you to use language that you feel comfortable with, but this chapter covers the basics of gynaecological anatomy, so that you know the correct terminology, should you need it.

Figures 1.1 and 1.2 show the external and internal gynaecological organs.

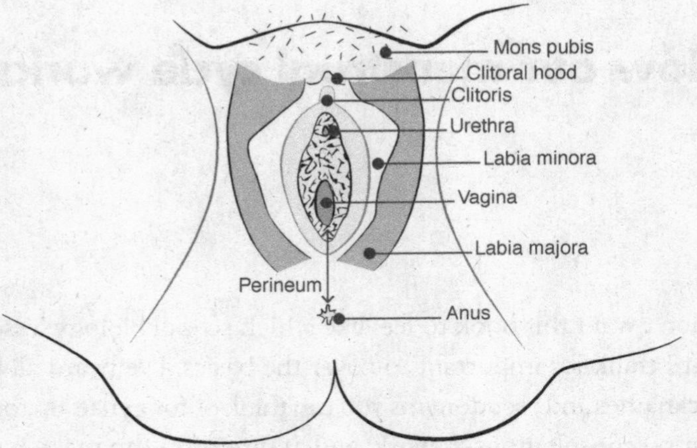

Figure 1.1. *A woman's external genitalia.*

External gynaecological anatomy

The vulva

The term 'vulva' derives from the Latin word for 'wrapper', and is used to refer to the external genitalia (the area that is visible from the outside). It contains the following structures:

Mons pubis – this is the spongy, fatty tissue covering the front of the pubic bone. The skin here is very sensitive and contains a lot of touch receptors. It is therefore covered with pubic hair, which provides some protection to the sensitive skin below, and also collects pheromones, which are the chemicals that play a role in sexual attraction.

Clitoris and clitoral hood – Many people don't realise that the clitoral head, a pea-sized structure sitting in front of the urethral opening, is only a tiny part of the clitoris. It is incredibly sensitive and therefore covered by a piece of skin called the clitoral hood. The whole clitoris is, in fact, shaped like a wishbone, with two legs that extend down either side underneath the surface of the labia minora. The legs are made of the same kind of tissue as a penis, which can become engorged and erect during sexual arousal.

Urethral opening – The urethra is the tube that connects the bladder to the outside, allowing drainage of urine. It has a similar name to the ureter, which is the tube higher up that connects the kidney to the bladder. During sexual arousal the tissue surrounding the urethral opening swells slightly: this is thought to be a protective feature in a bid to reduce the passage of bacteria up into the urethra during sex. Women are more prone to getting urinary tract infections (UTIs) than men since the urethra is much shorter, at about 5cm, compared to the 20cm urethra found in men.

Skene's glands, aka periurethral glands – These are the female version of the prostate gland. They produce a small amount of fluid, which provides some antibacterial protection from UTIs. They are also responsible for female ejaculation.

Vaginal opening and hymen – This is the entrance to the vagina. Just inside the vaginal opening is the hymen, which is a thin membrane of tissue that may be ring-shaped or half-moon-shaped. It's not known to have any specific biological function. The hymen can tear upon vaginal penetration, with tampon use or even during exercise, so the presence or absence of a hymen is not a reliable indicator of whether you've ever been sexually active. In about 1 in 2,000 women, this membrane extends across the entire vaginal opening, blocking it off, which is a condition called imperforate hymen. This is often diagnosed during the teenage years, usually because a girl's periods have not started, although these girls often report cyclical lower abdominal pain, because their hormones are working normally and the uterus is thickening and shedding its lining in the usual fashion, but the blood is trapped in the vagina behind the hymen and therefore cannot flow out. A relatively simple operation will remove this blockage.

Bartholin's glands – These sit next to the vaginal opening. They produce a mucus-like discharge, which reduces friction but may occasionally block the opening of the gland, resulting in the formation of a cyst, which if infected can form an abscess. This is incredibly painful. While some cysts can burst on their own, most need to be treated with antibiotics, as well as a small operation to drain the abscess in many cases. The idea of having an operation in that area sounds painful, I know, but the look of relief on my patients' faces afterwards tells me it's nothing compared to the abscess itself when it is at its worst.

Labia majora – The outer lips. The majora are made up of fatty tissue that cushions the delicate tissues of the external genitalia. These two skin folds are usually slightly darker than the surrounding skin. (In male fetuses, this area of the anatomy develops into the scrotum.)

Labia minora – These are the fleshy internal lips. They protect the urethral and vaginal openings. They can be various shades of pink, red, brown or black: they darken after puberty, and will change colour over a woman's lifetime. They meet at the front of the vulva in front of the clitoris and divide and spread down each side of the vulva. They are rarely symmetrical in size or shape, and it is quite normal for your labia minora to be visible below your labia majora.

Perineum – This is the region between the vaginal opening and the anus.

Internal gynaecological anatomy

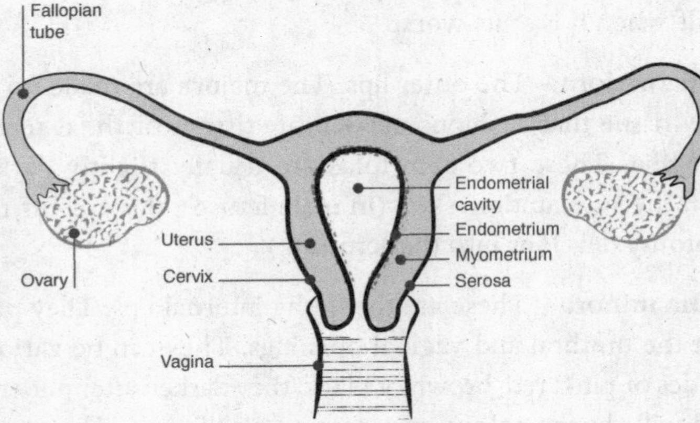

Figure 1.2. *Internal gynaecological anatomy.*

The vagina

The vagina is an elastic, muscular tube that can expand in length and width. In its relaxed state the walls of the vagina sit next to each other, keeping the vagina closed. The walls have small ridges called 'rugae', which contribute to its ability to expand and shrink back down. The vagina is not lined with skin, but instead with what is called a 'mucosa' – this is similar to the tissue that lines the inside of your mouth, and it is able to secrete fluid to maintain a moist environment. During sexual arousal, an increase in the blood flow to the vagina increases the amount of fluid that it releases, to provide lubrication. Vaginal discharge is an umbrella term to refer to fluid that comes from the vagina. The type of discharge that's present the rest of the time and is not related to arousal is mostly produced by the cervix; this is discussed later in this section.

The vagina is also very sensitive to oestrogen. During times of high oestrogen the tissue will be thicker, more plump, and tends to feel less dry or irritated. During times of low oestrogen, including early in the menstrual cycle and particularly after the menopause, vaginal tissue will be thinner and can feel quite dry, and often itchy and sensitive. The vagina is not sterile; it is designed to have a resident bacterial population, termed 'the vaginal microbiota'. These help to keep an acidic environment and provide some degree of protection from infections, including thrush, caused by yeasts, viruses such as the human papillomavirus (HPV), and sexually transmitted infections (STIs) such as chlamydia. Two things are very damaging to the normal bacterial population in your vagina: smoking, and washing your vagina, particularly with feminine hygiene washes. Although these are often pH-balanced, they wash away the good bacteria, *Lactobacillus*, and allow unpleasant bacteria to thrive. The result is itching, irritation and often a bad odour, so if these are the very reason you're using such products, I strongly encourage you to stop using them and I predict you will see a dramatic improvement. It's totally normal for your vulva and vagina to have a smell.

The uterus

The uterus, which is also known as the womb, is a muscular pear-shaped structure that sits very low down in the pelvis, at the top of your vagina. It's about 7–8cm from top to bottom and 5cm side to side on average. It may be marginally bigger in women who have had a baby than in those who have not. It also shrinks after the menopause. I frequently describe the uterus to patients as an upside-down wine bottle, with the larger, upper part representing the body of the uterus. It contains a cavity known as the endometrial cavity, and the narrower neck of the bottle represents the cervix, also referred to as 'the neck of the womb'.

The uterus has three layers. From the inside to the outside, these are the endometrium, myometrium and serosa. The endometrium lines the endometrial cavity, or the inside of the uterus. This is the layer that builds up throughout the menstrual cycle and is shed as a period. The endometrium is at its thinnest at the start of the menstrual cycle, and over the next 2 weeks it thickens up with the progressive rise in oestrogen levels. (The menstrual cycle is shown in Figure 2.1 on page 27.)

The myometrium is a thick layer of smooth muscle that contracts in a wave-like fashion during labour. It also contracts during your period to help shed the endometrium and allow this lining and the blood to escape through the cervix and out into the vagina at this time – this is what's happening when you experience period pain. In addition, the uterus isn't terribly fond of being touched, and may react by contracting and causing a similar period-like pain after deep penetrative sex, having cervical screening (which used to be known as a smear test), or similar.

The external layer is called the serosa. This is a slippery, smooth tissue that helps the uterus to glide without friction over the other pelvic organs.

The cervix

The cervix is the exit from, and entrance to, the uterus. There is a small tunnel through the middle of the cervix, called the cervical canal. The cervix opens during labour up to 10cm to allow the birth of a baby. It also softens and opens slightly during your period, to allow the blood to escape. The cervix has a very important job in protecting you from infections, by producing discharge that contains antibacterial and anti-viral compounds, as well as playing host to a healthy bacterial population. (The word 'discharge' is often thought to indicate something that is unclean or unhealthy, but in fact discharge is entirely normal and important for the above reasons. It also acts as a lubricant.) The inside of the cervix contains glands that produce and release this discharge, the texture of which changes throughout the menstrual cycle, based on the hormonal changes that you experience. Right after your period you might feel quite dry and there's very little vaginal fluid, but after a few days you may notice more of it, and it is often creamy in texture. As you move towards ovulation it will become much thinner, clear and eventually like egg white in texture, at which point it will be quite stretchy and stringy. This type of fluid is designed to help sperm travel through the cervix up into the uterus so it can meet and fertilise an egg. After ovulation the fluid once again becomes sticky, thick and sometimes slightly clumpy in nature. There is a reduction in the amount of discharge produced after the menopause, due to a reduction in oestrogen levels, and this can result in vaginal dryness, irritation, and pain during sex. However, none of these are things that you need to put up with. If you're experiencing any of these you should see your GP, who can discuss the use of vaginal oestrogen creams or tablets or vaginal lubricants, all of which can be very helpful.

Cervical ectropion

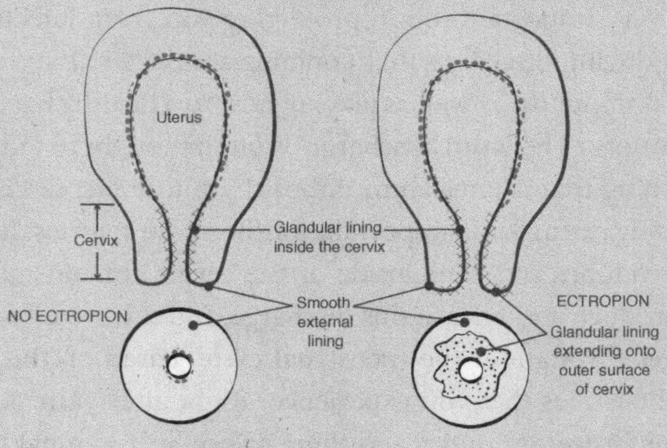

Figure 1.3: *Cervical ectropion.*

Normally the cervix has a smooth lining on the outside, with a slightly rougher, more fragile lining inside, where all the good protective discharge is made. In cervical ectropion, this lining also grows on the outside of the cervix (Figure 1.3). It is sometimes referred to as cervical erosion, but I'm not a fan of this term because it sounds like something has eaten away at your cervix, which is quite the opposite of the truth. In fact, ectropion happens because the cervix is effectively pushing out to expose those inner cells.

It's most common to find cervical ectropion in pregnant women, or women taking oestrogen-containing hormonal contraception, but some women have it for no specific reason. It's least commonly seen in women taking progestogen-only types of contraception, and after the menopause.

Ectropion causes increased amounts of vaginal discharge, bleeding after sex, and bleeding in between your periods. This bleeding happens because the tissue is fragile and can bleed at the slightest touch. There might be a few spots of blood, or enough to need to use a pad, and on occasions women describe bedroom scenes like a horror film after sex. Not what anyone wants to have to deal with when you'd much rather be having a cuddle!

You may also have no symptoms at all. You may happen to find out that you have ectropion during a routine smear test or speculum examination, during which it's seen by the person doing the test or examination.

Apart from the bleeding symptoms and/or discharge, cervical ectropion is harmless and does not increase your risk of cancer, fertility/pregnancy issues, etc.

In my experience, a lot of women are happy to leave it alone once they understand what it is and that it's nothing sinister, but many – understandably – want something to be done about it due to troublesome symptoms. In this case you can discuss a procedure to seal off the fragile tissue using either silver nitrate or a heated surgical instrument under local anaesthetic, to burn away the tissue or remove it entirely.

Fallopian tubes

There are two fallopian tubes, one coming from each upper, outer angle of the uterus. These link the ovary to the uterus, and eggs travel from the ovary into the uterus down the fallopian tubes. These tubes have a fluffy-looking end which contains little 'fingers' that help to pick up an egg from the ovary. It is then sucked into the tube and swept along by even tinier little finger-like projections called cilia, which sweep the egg along towards the uterus. If an egg is fertilised, this usually happens in the middle of the fallopian tube, and this fertilised egg continues its journey along the tube and into the uterus, where it will – hopefully – implant. About 50% of naturally fertilised eggs do not implant,[2] and those that don't cannot result in a pregnancy.

A pregnancy that implants anywhere other than inside the uterine cavity is called an ectopic pregnancy; 95% of these happen inside the fallopian tube. Unfortunately, an ectopic pregnancy cannot survive to become a healthy pregnancy; it needs to be treated. If left untreated, it can become a life-threatening emergency, because it can cause the fallopian tube to burst, resulting in massive internal bleeding. Many women who have had an ectopic pregnancy go on to have a healthy pregnancy, even after the removal of one fallopian tube. Interestingly, we know from women who have had one tube removed that it's possible for a tube to pick up an egg from either ovary. We know this because we see women who have had, for example, the left tube removed, but then have a healthy pregnancy which we can see has come from the left ovary, based on the fact that the left ovary contains a corpus luteum, which is a progesterone-secreting structure that can be seen in the ovulating ovary early in pregnancy.

While I have both fallopian tubes, when I got pregnant with my non-identical twins (which occurs as a result of two separate fertilised eggs), we could see that both eggs had come from the left ovary, which contained two corpus lutea, compared to the right ovary, which didn't contain any.

If both fallopian tubes are removed, or they are both damaged/blocked, you would need to have in vitro fertilisation (IVF) to become pregnant. There is no effective method to unblock fallopian tubes.

Ovaries

Women have two ovaries. These are not actually attached to the fallopian tubes, but sit very close by. They are suspended between two ligaments: one attaches the ovary to the side of your pelvis, and the other attaches the ovary to the side of your uterus. Ovaries contain eggs: women are born with their entire lifetime supply of eggs. At birth a woman has 2 million to 4 million eggs. Only about 1% of these make it to the point of being released. However, this doesn't mean that you have millions of eggs left behind. The eggs exist in an immature state. After you start your periods, every month hundreds of eggs start the maturation process to get ready to be released. This process takes several months, and the ovary creates a very efficient production line, ensuring that there are always eggs at various states of maturation to provide a mature egg for release each month. The eggs develop within follicles, which are small fluid-filled sacs, also known as cysts, that grow throughout the maturation process. You may have heard of ovarian cysts and think they are a bad thing, but making small ovarian cysts is completely normal, healthy, and part of the usual function of your ovaries. Follicles can grow to about 3cm in size, but the other types of ovarian cyst (discussed below) can become much bigger. Most follicles die away during the early maturation process, along with the eggs that they contain, but at the start of every menstrual cycle about ten maturing follicles are chosen as potentials for ovulation. These continue to mature until one is ultimately chosen to be the dominant follicle, which is the one destined for release at ovulation, which happens around 3 weeks after the start of your period and about one week before your next period, assuming you have a 28-day cycle (this is discussed on pages 26–31).

In addition to egg storage and release, the ovaries produce several important hormones, including oestrogens, progesterone, testosterone, inhibin and relaxin.

During a woman's fertile years the ovaries are around 3–4cm in size, and after the menopause the ovaries shrink to about 0.5–1cm in size. At this point in time they're no longer maturing and releasing eggs, but they still make very small amounts of oestrogen, with fat tissue and the adrenal glands becoming the main source of oestrogen production after menopause.

Ovarian cysts

A cyst is a fluid-filled sac. Remember that we all have cysts on our ovaries because it's how they release an egg. The egg lives in a follicle, which is a tiny cyst. It must grow and eventually burst to release the egg, which is then captured by the fallopian tube and transported into the uterus. A follicle usually grows up to about 3cm; if we're being very strict with the terminology, anything over 3cm can be referred to as a cyst. 'Functional' ovarian cysts form as part of the ovulation process and account for about 50% of all ovarian cysts. There are:

Simple cysts – Basically an oversized follicle that didn't realise it was time to stop growing and kept getting bigger, becoming a simple cyst. They have a fairly thin wall, are filled with clear fluid, and usually disappear on their own in a few months.

Corpus luteum cysts – The corpus luteum is the 'shell' of the egg that gets left behind. It pumps out progesterone, which dissolves away if you don't get pregnant in that cycle. If it doesn't, it can fill with fluid and form a cyst. They can bleed into themselves, which can be painful. This is described as a haemorrhagic corpus luteum cyst. This is not the same thing as an endometrioma (see below), and does not mean you have endometriosis.

Other types of common benign (non-cancerous) cysts that are not related to ovulation include:

Dermoid cysts – These are often described as 'cysts with teeth and hair'. They have the potential to develop into any kind of body cell, which is why they can contain hair, teeth, bone, fat cells, etc. If you're in any way squeamish, I wouldn't search Google Images for this term . . . Dermoid cysts don't disappear on their own because they contain solid tissue that can't dissolve away. That said, if you have a dermoid cyst, it doesn't always need to be removed. It could be observed by ultrasound, depending on the size, the symptoms you're having, and various other factors. Your doctor will be able to talk to you about this. There is a 1% risk of a dermoid cyst containing cancerous cells.

Endometriomas (aka chocolate cysts) – These are not as nice as they sound. They are described this way because they contain old, semi-digested blood that is brown. If you have an endometrioma, this means that you have endometriosis, which is discussed on pages 86–107.

Polycystic ovaries – This is diagnosed by ultrasound. This means there are 20 or more small follicles (tiny developing eggs) on your ovaries. Being told that your ovaries 'look polycystic' does not automatically mean that you have polycystic ovarian syndrome (PCOS). Your ovaries don't need removing, and this does not increase your risk of having the other types of cysts mentioned.

While most cysts are benign, some can be cancerous, and a doctor may suspect this based on their appearance on a scan. Some are described as 'borderline', which means they contain abnormal cells that have a small risk of turning into a cancer. The size of a cyst doesn't always correlate with the chance of it being cancerous. Some of the biggest cysts I've removed have been completely benign.

Symptoms of an ovarian cyst include pain, pressure symptoms on your bladder, feeling bloated or a lump in your stomach, but often they're found on an ultrasound scan that is being performed for other reasons. In a small number of cases they can present suddenly with sudden, very severe lower abdominal pain, which might be due to them bursting (a cyst accident) or twisting (torsion), so that the cyst blocks off the blood supply to the ovary. The risk of this is very small, but the larger the cyst, the higher this becomes. Cysts don't usually cause changes to your periods.

Surgery may be required to remove a cyst. This is covered on page 275, although not all cysts need to be removed; some will disappear on their own.

Chapter 2

What is a 'normal' period?

A period is the vaginal bleeding that occurs when the endometrium (the internal lining of the uterus) sheds away. There is blood, mixed with mucus and old endometrial lining. Contrary to what some people say, your period is not a way of 'detoxifying your body'. While our endometrium is pretty incredible, given its ability to develop, shed and regenerate on a regular basis, it doesn't have any method of selecting toxic substances for removal (unlike the liver and kidneys, where detoxification actually takes place). Your body has a period quite simply because you didn't get pregnant, which might seem strange given that most woman are not trying to get pregnant the majority of the time. Quite the opposite, in fact! A period can also be referred to as menstruation, which is a word derived from the Latin word for 'month' and the Greek word for 'moon', because the menstrual cycle was thought to be connected to the lunar cycle, as they both lasted about a month. The terminology around periods and menstruation can be a little confusing, so I've added a glossary below of all the terms that you might hear.

Glossary of period-related medical terms

- Abnormal uterine bleeding (AUB) – any bleeding from the uterus in a non-pregnant woman or girl that is abnormal in amount, frequency, duration and/or regularity.
- Amenorrhoea – the absence of a menstrual period. This may be temporary or permanent.
    - Primary amenorrhoea – failure to establish menstruation by age 15 with normal secondary sexual characteristics including pubic hair growth and breast development) or by age 13 with absence of secondary sexual characteristics.
    - Secondary amenorrhoea – periods that have stopped for 3–6 months or more.
- Anovulation – when an egg is not released during a menstrual cycle.
- Dysmenorrhoea – cramping pains in the lower abdomen before and/or during a period.
    - Primary dysmenorrhoea – no underlying cause found.

- Secondary dysmenorrhoea – due to an underlying condition, e.g. endometriosis.
- Dyspareunia – pain during or after sexual intercourse.
    - Deep dyspareunia – pain related to deeper penetration.
    - Superficial dyspareunia – pain limited to the vulva or vagina.
- Flooding – a sudden gush of menstrual blood.
- Intermenstrual bleeding – bleeding in between your periods.
- Menarche – the first menstrual period.
- Menopause – when your periods have stopped permanently for 12 months or more.
- Menorrhagia – heavy menstrual bleeding.
- Menstrual cycle – a complex sequence of hormonal changes and structural changes to the ovaries and uterus that occur to prepare for a possible pregnancy. The first day of your menstrual cycle is the first day of a menstrual period, and the last day is the day before the next menstrual period.
- Menstruation – vaginal bleeding occurring as part of the menstrual cycle, also known as a menstrual period.

- Ovulation – when an egg is released from the ovary.
- Perimenopause – the time leading up to the menopause.
- Postcoital bleeding – vaginal bleeding after sexual intercourse.
- Spotting – very light vaginal bleeding which may be pink or brown, but not enough to need to use period products such as a pad or tampon.

The term 'menstrual cycle' refers to the length of time from the start of one period until the day before the next period (Figure 2.1). During this time, a complex sequence of hormonal changes takes place in order to prepare the body for a potential pregnancy. The start of your bleeding marks the start of a new cycle, also known as Day 1. All the textbooks and health literature talk about a 'typical 28-day cycle', but only about 15% of us actually have this classic 28-day cycle.[3] A normal cycle is between 21 and 35 days.

While the period is the part of the cycle that gets the most focus, there is a great deal of action going on behind the scenes for the remainder of the cycle, and I'll take you through that now.

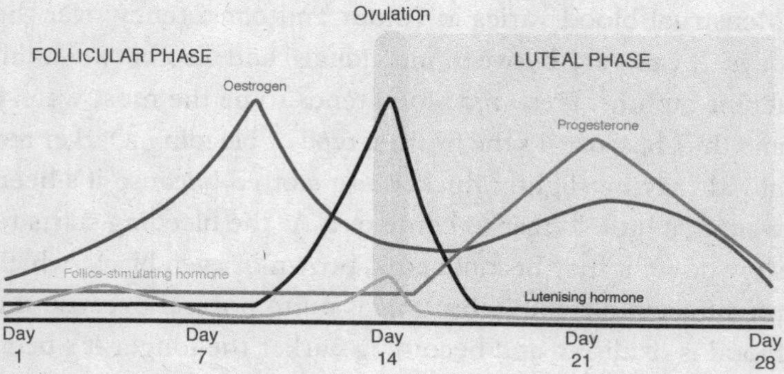

Figure 2.1. *The menstrual cycle.*

A menstrual cycle

The follicular phase

This first phase of the menstrual cycle starts with the first day of your period – also known as Day 1. The follicular phase lasts from Day 1 to Day 13 (assuming you have a 28-day cycle). It's quite common to get a bit of spotting before your period starts, which means very light bleeding that isn't enough to need to use a period product such as a pad, tampon or menstrual cup. Day 1 should be the first day of proper bleeding that requires the use of a period product. Bleeding is typically at its heaviest on Day 2 and then will gradually slow down. A period lasts for an average of 5 days, but can range from 3–8 days.

Menstrual blood varies in colour and consistency over the days. It can vary between individuals, and also between different months. Fresh red blood tends to be the most watery and thin, because it's the freshest type of bleeding. Darker red blood may be slightly thicker and clotted because it's been waiting a little longer to come out. As the bleeding starts to slow down it may become pink, brown or even black, which might seem alarming, but this is quite normal because the blood is oxidising and becoming darker the longer it's been around, in the same way that the surface of a cut apple turns brown over time. I've seen social media posts about 'what the colour of your menstrual blood is telling you', but to be completely honest, I don't think there's any truth to it. I've never diagnosed anyone with a particular condition based on the colour of their blood. And if these articles are to be believed, I really ought to get myself to a gynaecologist based on the rainbow of colours I've seen coming out of my own vagina!

In addition, menstrual blood isn't just blood. In fact, it's been estimated that about 36% of your period is actual blood, and the remainder is the old endometrial cells that are shed, along with cervical and vaginal secretions.[4]

Clots are quite common, and occur as a result of a very normal process. As blood is shed from the uterus, it clots and needs to be broken down by chemicals called anticoagulants to become liquid again, to make it easier to pass through the cervix (which softens slightly during your period to facilitate this). The muscle layer of the uterus also contracts, like mini labour pains, to push the blood out. Some women who have very heavy periods with lots of clots will read this and think, 'Dr Anita, there's nothing mini about these pains!' And they're right. The more blood and clots there are to pass, the more intense the pain can be, because your uterus is trying very hard to evacuate everything. Clots should generally be no larger than a 50p piece. Large clots and/or passing a lot of clots can be a sign that the normal anticoagulation process is becoming overwhelmed, meaning your body is unable to break down the clots quickly enough because they're being produced in such abundance. This is a sign that you should see your GP so they can look for an underlying cause, offer treatment, and ensure that you're not becoming anaemic, which can soon happen if you have this kind of bleeding every time you have a period (see page 70).

While this is going on inside your uterus, there's also hard work going on behind the scenes. Follicle-stimulating hormone (FSH) is made in the pituitary gland in the brain: it makes your ovaries do exactly what it says on the tin: stimulate some follicles. Those that aren't released as eggs simply shrink away. After your period the endometrium will be at its thinnest. The developing follicles produce oestrogen, which causes the endometrium to be rebuilt, thicken and develop so that it is ready to accommodate a pregnancy. The rise in oestrogen also signals to the brain that it's time to ovulate, and for this a second hormone called luteinising hormone (LH) is required. There is a huge spike in LH levels 24–36 hours before ovulation, which is when the egg is released. LH is the hormone that is detected by ovulation prediction kits (OPKs: see page 37 for more info). I always describe LH to my patients as a big pin that comes along and pops the egg out of its sac.

The luteal phase

Ovulation marks the start of the luteal phase (which is Day 14 to Day 28, if you have a 28-day cycle). You can only ovulate once per menstrual cycle, but it's possible to release more than one egg when you ovulate. If each egg is fertilised by a different sperm, this produces non-identical twins (or triplets!). It's more common for older women to have non-identical twins because your body makes more FSH to stimulate the ovaries as your egg reserve starts to decline.

The luteal phase is so called because once the egg is released the structure left behind in your ovary is called the corpus luteum. Its role is to produce progesterone, which is the 'pro-gestational' or 'pro-pregnancy' hormone, responsible for maintaining an early pregnancy until the placenta is able to take over. Progesterone stops oestrogen from causing the endometrium to thicken any further and causes it to develop various properties that are necessary to sustain a pregnancy, including the formation of a complex network of blood vessels. Progesterone levels peak about 7 days after ovulation. If the corpus luteum isn't getting signals that there is actually a pregnancy to maintain, it starts to die away, and progesterone levels start to fall as a result. Oestrogen levels also peak around the same time as progesterone, and the combination of these two hormones at high levels can result in premenstrual symptoms. Due to this drop in oestrogen and progesterone, your body is no longer able to sustain the endometrium, and this results in the upper two-thirds of the endometrium shedding away within the next 7 days, which is your period. The drop in progesterone also triggers the formation of prostaglandins, which are chemical messengers that cause the uterus to contract. This helps the body to expel the endometrial lining – and this contraction is also responsible for period pains.

I'm aware that I keep referring to pregnancy when I talk about the menstrual cycle, which might be irritating if pregnancy isn't on your radar. And if you've been trying to get pregnant but you're having problems, this might be incredibly frustrating to read. I'm sorry for that. I've included some fertility resources on page 318, and please contact your GP if you are having trouble in this area. However, your menstrual cycle exists purely to prepare your body for a pregnancy.

Bowel changes during your period

Also known as 'period poops'!

As if having a period wasn't enough to deal with, about one-third of us are also troubled by bowel symptoms at the same time, including bloating, diarrhoea or constipation, although this figure increases to about 50% if you have irritable bowel syndrome (IBS). Studies show that these symptoms are often worse on Day 1 of bleeding.[5]

This fluctuation in symptoms relates to the impact of oestrogen and progesterone levels on the gut, the production of prostaglandins (the chemicals that cause contractions of the uterine muscle, which results in shedding of the womb lining, causing period pain) that alter gut motility, and the influence of hormonal fluctuations on the gut microbiome. It has also been suggested that stress related to having your period can result in bowel symptoms due to the gut–brain connection – in the same way that you might experience diarrhoea if you're nervous or anxious about something.

There are no sure-fire ways to prevent this. Some people find that avoiding certain foods can help, but this is very individual so keep an eye out for any foods that you find make symptoms better or worse.

Endometriosis can affect your bowel and may cause pain when you open your bowels. This may occur only during your period or throughout your menstrual cycle, and can worsen at the time of your period. It can also cause blood in your stools during your period, and is a reason to see your doctor. Endometriosis is covered in more depth on page 86 onwards.

Other issues around your period

Anovulatory cycles

Have you ever had a period that came at completely the wrong time, and the bleeding and your premenstrual syndrome (PMS) symptoms were different to normal? Chances are, you had an **anovulatory** cycle.

As you can see, it's ovulation that determines the timing of your period. This is a necessary step for progesterone production and the start of the second phase of the menstrual cycle: the luteal phase. If you're ovulating reliably, the timing of your period should also be reliable. Several factors (such as stress, travel across time zones, illness, a significant change in diet or exercise) can change the timing of ovulation, either bringing it forward, making your period arrive earlier than expected, or more commonly pushing it back, resulting in your period being more than fashionably late.

But these factors can also stop you from ovulating altogether. Not ovulating is called anovulation, and it's particularly common if you have hypothalamic amenorrhoea (page 148) or polycystic ovary syndrome (PCOS) (page 125). It's also very common when you start your periods and end them, which is why your periods may be irregular to start with, and then again prior to the menopause.

Do women's menstrual cycles synchronise if they live together?

Unfortunately, this is not true. This concept first came about in 1971, and is called the McClintock effect, named after the psychologist who wrote the first research study on this topic.[6] The study was based in a college dormitory and suggested that the menstrual cycles of women who were room-mates and close friends synced up. However, the methods used in the study have been called into question, and there have been multiple further studies since then that have tried to replicate this but none of them came to the same conclusion, so while it seems like a nice idea, cycle syncing doesn't appear to be a real phenomenon.

When you don't release an egg, minimal progesterone is produced, so you don't get the natural drop in progesterone to stimulate the lining of your uterus to shed. So how do you bleed after an anovulatory cycle? Oestrogen causes your uterine lining to thicken, and progesterone usually helps to sustain it and develop it so it can support a pregnancy. Without progesterone, oestrogen does its best to maintain the uterine lining, but it eventually fails and the lining begins to fall away as a period. If you've got plenty of oestrogen your period might be heavier than normal because your body has had longer than normal to grow the uterine lining. Some women who have anovulatory cycles can have low oestrogen and therefore their uterine lining will be pretty scanty so the resulting period could be very light.

Periods on the pill

The most common schedule for using the combined oral contraceptive pill (COCP) is to take it for 21 days, during which time you'll have a consistent level of oestrogen and progesterone, and then have 7 pill-free days. The abrupt withdrawal of these hormones will cause bleeding to start in 3–4 days, mimicking the natural decline in oestrogen and progesterone that occurs in a normal menstrual cycle (Figure 2.1), so sometimes the period you get while on the pill is called a 'withdrawal bleed' rather than a period. This can be confusing because it's essentially the same thing. In both situations the bleeding is happening because of a drop in hormone levels, but one is due to natural hormone production and the other is due to not taking the tablets. The COCP is covered in more detail on pages 98–9.

If you're using the progesterone-only pill (POP), an implant, injection or the Mirena® IUS (intrauterine system), you may still continue to have periods, but the timing of your periods won't be controlled in the same way as it is with the COCP, because you're using these contraceptives all the time. If you are using hormonal contraception and your periods stop, this is not dangerous, because the progesterone is protecting your endometrium, keeping it relatively thin. But if you're not having periods and you are not taking any external progesterone, you could be at risk of developing a condition called endometrial hyperplasia (see page 139), due to a lack of progesterone and its protective effect on the endometrium.

The copper coil does not contain any hormones, so you'll still have your usual menstrual cycle.

Ovulation

Many women are confused about ovulation – when does this happen in their cycle? How do you know if you're ovulating? How much pain is normal? – so this section discusses these issues and more.

How to know when you are ovulating

Some women like to look out for signs of ovulation to understand where they are in their cycle, as reassurance that everything is working as it should, or because they're trying to get pregnant. Here's how you can find out if, and when, ovulation is happening:

Ovulation discharge – This is a very thin, watery discharge that then becomes incredibly stretchy, with an egg-white consistency. This helps the sperm to get through the cervix so that it can meet and fertilise an egg.

Changes in basal body temperature – Your basal body temperature dips just before ovulation and rises by up to 1°C afterwards. You should take your temperature first thing in the morning, before you get out of bed, and make a note of it so you can see changes over time.

Ovulation prediction kits (OPKs) – These are home urine tests, taken like a pregnancy test. They measure LH in your urine, so an OPK will be positive about 24–36 hours before ovulation. These kits don't confirm that you actually ovulated, but they tell you there's been an LH surge. (A word of warning: If you have PCOS, OPKs can be quite unreliable because you may have a higher baseline LH level than someone without PCOS, and have multiple small LH surges, meaning the test can be positive but you're not actually about to ovulate.)

Blood tests – You can test your progesterone level to determine whether ovulation actually happened. We typically refer to this as 'Day 21 progesterone', because with a 28-day cycle progesterone should be at its peak on Day 21, or 7 days before your period. If your cycle isn't 28 days, you need to subtract 7 days from the total length of your cycle to work out the right time for you to take the test. For example, if your cycle is 31 days, 31 − 7 = 24, so you'd take it on Day 24. If progesterone levels are high, this shows you have ovulated. If they're low, you either didn't ovulate or you ovulated at a different time to when you expected, so you'll need to repeat the test at a different time. Your doctor will help you work this out.

Ultrasound follicle tracking – This is a series of ultrasound scans that can be performed to predict the timing of ovulation based on the number and size of follicles present in the ovaries, along with the thickness of the endometrium.

Note: If you are taking the COCP or using a contraceptive implant or injection you will not ovulate – these contraceptives work by stopping ovulation. Some women on the POP or using the Mirena® will still ovulate, so may notice some of these changes.

Ovulation pain

Ovulation pain affects about one-third of women and girls. It can be experienced as a mild pain or cramp in your lower abdomen, sometimes on one side, sometimes in the middle. It happens at the time of ovulation, usually around Day 10–14, and lasts 12–24 hours.

No one is really sure why it happens, but it's thought to be due to the release of prostaglandins, which are chemicals that cause tiny muscles around the follicles in the ovary to contract, to help release the egg. This could explain why some women feel pain before the egg is actually released.[7]

Over-the-counter painkillers, heat (such as a hot water bottle on the affected area) and keeping mobile can all help to ease the discomfort. If the pain is very severe, you should consider seeing your GP, who will assess you to rule out any other causes. If they don't think there is any other cause of the pain, they could prescribe you the COCP, which works by stopping ovulation. The POP is also an option, but it's slightly less effective because its primary mechanism is not to stop ovulation (although it does so in 60–97% of women, depending on the type of progesterone it contains).

Ovulation pain does not indicate anything about the health or function of your ovaries.

Anecdotally, many women tell me that they started to experience ovulation pain after the birth of their first child, or it started to get worse then. I'm not aware of any scientific studies that have looked at this, but if it happens to you, you're not alone.

Ovulation bleeding

At the time of ovulation there is a momentary drop in oestrogen levels which can trigger a little bleeding or spotting. This is quite normal, and not a sign of anything sinister. This occurs in about 3% of cycles.[8] If you're experiencing heavy bleeding around the time of ovulation, or bleeding in between your periods, please speak to your doctor, as there are other things that could be causing this bleeding, including infections, polyps, fibroids and, in rare cases, cancers of the cervix or endometrium.

Breast changes throughout the menstrual cycle

Your breasts contain oestrogen and progesterone receptors and therefore change throughout the menstrual cycle.

Oestrogen stimulates growth of the milk ducts, which are the passageways through which milk travels to the nipple. After ovulation, there is a rise in progesterone. This prepares your breasts for a potential pregnancy by prompting growth of the milk lobules, which are like tiny bunches of grapes that produce the milk that then feeds into the ducts. At this time your breasts can feel very swollen, sore and lumpy. Once your period starts you should begin to feel relief rather rapidly, and your breasts will begin to shrink down and start to feel softer.

If you're taking hormonal contraception or HRT you may find that your breasts are slightly larger than usual, and they can be tender or more sensitive. Sometimes this is temporary, settling down after a few months, but if you find the change too difficult to deal with you should speak to your doctor and discuss a potential change of medication.

Checking your breasts

It's estimated that 40% of breast cancers are detected by self-examination. The NHS Breast Screening Programme has five tips for breast awareness, which are:

1. Know what's normal for you.
2. Look at your breasts and feel them.
3. Know what changes to look for (see below).
4. Report any changes to your GP without delay.
5. Attend breast screening if you're aged 50 to 70 (From https://www.nhs.uk/common-health-questions/lifestyle/how-should-i-check-my-breasts/)

The best time to check your breasts is about a week after your period starts because this is when your breasts are likely to be at their least tender or swollen, but you can still check them at other times of your cycle to understand the normal changes that your breasts go through, because this will be different for everyone.

Any of the following should prompt a trip to the GP:

- A change in the size, outline or shape of your breast.
- A change in the look or feel of the skin on your breast, such as puckering or dimpling, a rash or redness.
- A new lump, swelling, thickening or bumpy area in one breast or armpit that was not there before.

- A discharge of fluid from either nipple.
- A change in nipple position, such as your nipple being pulled in or pointing differently.
- A rash (like eczema), crusting, scaly or itchy skin, or redness on or around your nipple.
- Any discomfort or pain in one breast, particularly if it's a new pain and does not go away. (Note: Pain is a very rare symptom of breast cancer.)

www.coppafeel.org is a brilliant website that contains information about breasts and how to check them.

Menarche to the menopause: the first to the last period and beyond

Menarche

Menarche means 'first menstrual period'. The average age for this to happen in the UK is 12.9 years.[9] Girls usually have their first period 2–3 years after their breasts start to develop. However, starting your periods aged from 9 to 15 is considered within the normal range. Studies have shown that this age has decreased over time: in 1840, girls started their periods at the age of 17, on average.[10] The timing of menarche is thought to be partly genetic but also related to environmental factors that start before a child is even born. Smoking during pregnancy and pre-eclampsia (a pregnancy complication where you develop high blood pressure with protein in your urine) have been linked to earlier age at first period, as have greater childhood height and body weight.[11] When you start your periods has also been linked to when your periods will end: having your first period before the age of 11 is linked to having an earlier menopause.[12]

Starting your periods can be a difficult time, particularly because periods are often unpredictable in both timing and nature. They can be painful and heavy. It's not uncommon to experience occasional vomiting and fainting when periods start: these are in response to the prostaglandins that cause period pain, as well as to the pain itself. I want to reassure you that periods do usually settle down and get easier, but if your period – or your daughter's period – is having a significant impact on daily life then please see your GP. You don't have to suffer in silence. There are various treatment options, hormonal and non-hormonal, and it may also be worth checking for anaemia too if periods are consistently very heavy.

Primary amenorrhoea

Primary amenorrhoea is defined as:

- periods that have not started by the age of 13, and you have not developed breasts or pubic hair; or

- periods that have not started by the age of 15, but you have developed breasts and/or pubic hair.

If this is the case, you should see your GP, who can start investigations. Primary amenorrhoea occurs in less than 1% of women, while secondary amenorrhoea may be experienced by about 4% of women of normal menstruating age.[13]

There are numerous causes of primary amenorrhoea, many of which are incredibly rare. Here are some of the most common causes:

- Constitutional delay – No abnormality is found, but a girl is developing at a slightly slower pace than average.
- Anatomical variations, including:
    - Imperforate hymen (see page 8).
    - Mayer–Rokitansky–Küster–Hauser (MRKH) syndrome – This results in an underdeveloped vagina and no uterus. The ovaries usually develop and function normally, so women born with this condition have the option to harvest their eggs to use in an IVF pregnancy, which would be carried by a surrogate. Many people I speak to are surprised to hear that surrogacy is legal in the UK. If you are considering this option, then this website may be useful: https://www.gov.uk/legal-rights-when-using-surrogates-

and-donors. MRKH syndrome is the second most common cause of primary amenorrhoea.

- Genetic conditions, including:
  - Turner syndrome – Humans normally have 46 chromosomes, two of which are sex chromosomes: XX develops into a female body and XY develops into a male body. People with Turner syndrome only have one sex chromosome, which is a single X. As a result, the ovaries do not develop or function normally. Turner syndrome occurs in about 1 in 2,000 women and is the most common cause of primary amenorrhoea.
- Hormonal conditions, including:
  - Congenital adrenal hyperplasia – This is a group of conditions caused by an inherited deficiency in some of the enzymes required to produce hormones in the adrenal gland.
- Ovarian conditions, including:
  - Premature menopause – This is rare, but it means that menopause has taken place before periods have even started.
  - Surgery, chemotherapy or radiotherapy-induced ovarian failure following treatment for childhood cancers.

Menopause and perimenopause

The menopause is the time in a woman's life when her periods stop. It can only be confirmed once a woman has had 12 months without a period, at which point she becomes postmenopausal. The exception to this rule is if a woman has had her ovaries surgically removed, in which case she would immediately become postmenopausal. This is called the surgical menopause and is discussed on pages 283–4.

The average age to go through the natural menopause is 51, and it usually happens somewhere between 45 and 55 years. Early menopause is defined as menopause before the age of 45, and it affects about 10% of women. Premature menopause, also referred to as primary ovarian insufficiency (POI) or premature ovarian failure (POF), is defined as menopause before the age of 40 years. This affects 1% of women overall, about 0.1% before the age of 30 and 0.01% before the age of 20 (see page 160). Multiple studies have shown that genetics play a factor in the timing of menopause, so it may be worth asking your mum when her menopause was, to get an idea of what you might expect. Environmental factors including smoking and night-shift work have been linked with an earlier menopausal age, and using the contraceptive pill and having a higher body mass index (BMI) with a slightly later menopause.

Menopause happens because the ovaries run out of eggs and stop producing oestrogen. The perimenopause is the phase leading up to the menopause. During this time your hormones will fluctuate as your egg supply dwindles, and this is when you may begin to experience menopausal symptoms and changes in your menstrual cycle. Periods can become irregular and unpredictable in timing or nature. A study has shown that the average age for this to occur is 47 or 48.[14] In the early phase of the perimenopause, your menstrual cycle may become shorter by 2–4 days: hormonal changes result in slightly earlier ovulation, leading to a shorter follicular phase. About 25% of women also begin to experience heavier bleeding because their oestrogen level becomes – paradoxically – higher, and progesterone is low. During the later phase of perimenopause, ovulation becomes rarer, your oestrogen level drops, periods may become much lighter and your cycle lengthens (up to around 60 days). Many women report missing periods until they eventually stop altogether. About 10% of women won't experience any of these changes in their cycle; their periods will just stop.

About 80–90% of women will experience some menopausal symptoms. These are largely related to the drop in oestrogen, with hot flushes and night sweats being the most common. Many are quite non-specific, yet troublesome, such as insomnia, memory loss, inability to concentrate, low mood, reduced libido, joint pain, headaches and palpitations. Many of the symptoms of the menopause are the same as the symptoms of depression, which unfortunately results in many women being misdiagnosed. Menopausal symptoms last an average of 7 years, and 25% of women describe their symptoms as 'severe' and 'debilitating'. While modifying your lifestyle might be helpful – for example, reducing your caffeine and alcohol intake, maintaining good sleep hygiene, eating well and exercising regularly – you may wish to consider the use of hormone replacement therapy (HRT) to reduce your symptoms. Your GP will be able to discuss HRT with you and prescribe it if it's appropriate. In some circumstances, such as if you've had cancer or have a complicated medical history, it might be more appropriate for you to be seen by a menopause specialist (this may be a GP, a gynaecologist or an endocrinologist – a doctor specialising in hormonal conditions – or a specialist nurse who has undertaken extra training in the provision of menopause care). If you cannot take HRT, or would prefer not to, other medications may help, depending on your symptoms and general health. While some women are misdiagnosed with depression during the menopause, I should point out here that some antidepressants can be useful during the menopause, especially to treat hot flushes, particularly in women who can't use HRT, so in some circumstances an antidepressant may be the correct medication for you, even if you're not depressed.

The menopause is getting so much more publicity these days, which is great – it's good to raise awareness of all the possible symptoms and encourage women to seek help if they need it. However, not every woman needs HRT – or any other form of medication – during the menopause, it depends how you feel. Also, you don't have to wait for your periods to stop to start taking HRT, and there's no time limit on how long you can use it.

Blood tests to diagnose the menopause are generally unhelpful over the age of 45, because hormone levels can change so much over a month. Instead, treatment is based on symptoms. There are a few exceptions to this rule, though, and here are a few circumstances in which checking FSH levels might be helpful:

- Women aged over 50 who are not having periods due to hormonal contraception.
- Women aged 40–45 with symptoms that suggest early menopause.
- Women aged under 40 with symptoms that suggest premature menopause.

Bleeding after the menopause

Vaginal bleeding after the menopause – also known as post-menopausal bleeding (PMB) – always requires medical attention. About 1 in 10 women will have some PMB, but just because it's common, this doesn't make it normal.

One of the best comments I've seen on social media was a reply to one of my posts about PMB from a woman who said that she'd realised, from my post, that PMB was not normal.

She was having PMB so she saw her GP, was diagnosed with endometrial cancer, and was recovering from a hysterectomy. I mean, wow! I don't claim to have saved her life, but I'm glad that my message was seen by the right person, and she was able to get the investigations and treatment she needed before her cancer spread.

Cancer is, of course, the number-one thing that patients and doctors worry about with PMB. If you report PMB to your GP, they will refer you to see a gynaecologist via the Two-Week Wait pathway, which is used for suspected cancer cases. While most cases of PMB are not cancer, it is something that we need to exclude. This is done by performing an internal examination, ultrasound scan and, if indicated, a hysteroscopy (see page 272).

Causes of bleeding include:

Endometrial cancer or hyperplasia – It's estimated that 10% of women with PMB will have endometrial cancer, and 15% will have endometrial hyperplasia.

Atrophic endometritis – A lack of oestrogen during the menopause causes the thin endometrium to become more prone to inflammation and infections, resulting in bleeding.

Atrophic vaginitis – A lack of oestrogen causes thinning of the vulval and vaginal skin, which can become very fragile and inflamed, making it prone to bleeding, even with minimal or no contact.

Endometrial or cervical polyps (see page 136).

Medications (e.g. HRT, blood thinners, tamoxifen).

Ovarian cancer – PMB is a rare symptom of ovarian cancer. This can be caused by the growth of a rare type of ovarian tumour that makes its own oestrogen, causing thickening of the endometrium, resulting in vaginal bleeding.

Cervical cancer – Approximately 40% of cases occur in women who have gone through the menopause, so it's very important that you attend cervical screening (smear test) regularly, no matter your age and level of sexual activity.

Vulva cancer – This is quite rare, with only about 1,000 cases per year in the UK.

Vaginal cancer – This is even more rare, with about 250 cases per year in the UK.

HRT and breast cancer

When I suggest to a patient that she considers taking HRT, a very common response is 'But isn't that going to increase my chance of breast cancer?'

The link between HRT and breast cancer has received a great deal of media attention, and the simple answer to this question is: there *is* an increased risk of breast cancer with the use of HRT, but no increased risk of dying from breast cancer. In addition, using HRT reduces all-cause mortality (the total number of deaths for any reason) and specifically heart-disease-related deaths, as well as reducing the risk of bone loss and fractures.

It's impossible to give anyone their personal risk of breast cancer, but the British Menopause Society has produced a helpful summary of the risks of breast cancer that I often use when discussing HRT with my patients.[15] I have summarised it here:

Per 1,000 women aged 50–59 in the UK population:

- Twenty-three will develop breast cancer over the next 5 years.
- Additional four cases with use of combined HRT (containing oestrogen and progesterone).
- Four fewer cases with use of oestrogen-only HRT (this is only suitable for women who have had a hysterectomy – see page 176).
- Additional four cases with use of combined oral contraceptive pill (containing oestrogen and progesterone).
- Additional five cases in women who drink two or more units of alcohol per day.
- Additional three cases in current smokers.
- Additional 23 cases in women with a BMI of 30 or more.

- Seven fewer cases in women who take more than 2.5 hours of moderate exercise per week.

As you can see, women can make several lifestyle changes to decrease their risk of breast cancer before considering whether HRT might be right from them.

No one wants to get breast cancer, and no doctor wants their patient to get breast cancer, but I think it's important to discuss these statistics to put them into perspective. If we don't, I believe that many women will dismiss HRT – a treatment that can have a profoundly positive impact on their quality of life. Ultimately, each person must feel comfortable about taking a medication, but I strongly believe that every woman deserves to have a personalised conversation with a healthcare professional about this.

Period products

There are an overwhelming number of products on the market, often referred to as 'feminine hygiene' or 'menstrual hygiene' items. I dislike the term 'hygiene' because it suggests that periods are dirty. They're not; they are a completely normal part of being female.

I'm frequently asked, 'What's the best thing to use?' I don't think there's one product that's better, safer, healthier, so I advise you to use whichever you feel most comfortable with. I'd like to reflect on the fact that having a choice about period products really is a luxury. Period poverty – the inability to afford period products – is not just something that happens in developing countries. A survey by Action Aid published in May 2022 showed that 12% of women in Britain have struggled to afford products for themselves or dependents over the past 6 months.[16] That's 1 in 8 women, many of whom reported using tissues instead of a pad/tampon, or keeping pads or tampons in for longer than they'd like.

Menstrual cups

These are reusable egg-cup-shaped devices made of silicone, latex or rubber. A menstrual cup (Figure 2.2) sits at the top of your vagina, just below your cervix, and collects blood as it comes out. Menstrual cups look a lot wider than a tampon, which might seem off-putting, but remember that your vagina is very elastic: it will be able to make space for a cup, and menstrual cups won't cause your vagina to stretch permanently. Learning to use them can take a bit of patience, and you have to be comfortable with putting your fingers into your vagina to insert and remove the cup – they don't come with an applicator, like a tampon does. Once the cup is in place, you shouldn't feel it. It can stay in for up to 12 hours, when it needs to be removed and rinsed before being reinserted. It should be cleaned with boiling water at the end of your period and before you start to use it for your next period. The cup stays in place by creating a vacuum which needs to be broken to remove the cup. This can be done by inserting your finger and thumb and pinching the base of the cup. You can usually feel that the vacuum has been broken, and then you can safely pull it out. It can be a skill to remove it without spilling anything, particularly when you're new to using cups, so I recommend trying it in the shower the first few times to avoid having to clean the bathroom floor afterwards. The Chartered Society of Physiotherapists has called for menstrual cup manufacturers to provide more in-depth safety advice on their use, due to concerns that the incorrect removal of menstrual cups might contribute to the risk of pelvic organ prolapse (see box below), due to women straining their pelvic floor muscles to push the cup down to remove it. Do not bear down or pull on the cup's stem to remove it, as this will put strain on your pelvic floor and the supporting pelvic ligaments. However, keep in mind that there are other things that can lead to the risk of prolapse, such as chronic cough or constipation. It's very unlikely that a menstrual cup by itself would cause a prolapse.

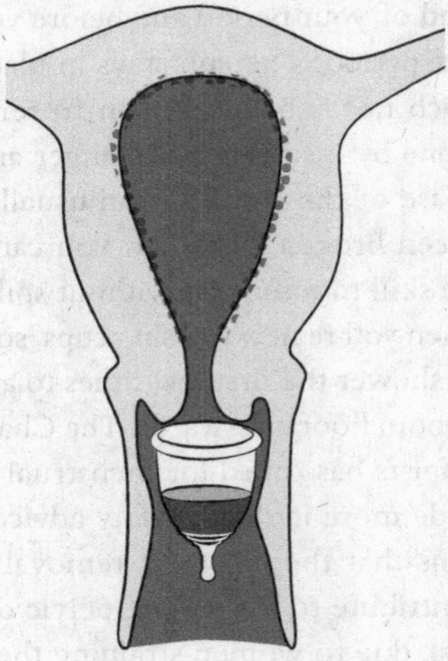

Figure 2.2. A *menstrual cup and where it is positioned.*

Another common question regarding menstrual cups is whether it's safe to use them with a contraceptive coil (a hormonal coil or a copper coil). Due to the slight vacuum effect exerted by menstrual cups, coils falling out seems to be associated with cup use, although the research on this is relatively scarce.[17] Coils can, of course, fall out if you don't use a menstrual cup. About 5% of coils fall out, and this is most common in the first 3 months after insertion.

I do know of women who have accidentally removed their coil using a menstrual cup. The problem is, once it's out, you can't put it back in. If you choose to use a cup with a coil, my best advice is to check your coil's strings by inserting a finger into your vagina at the end of your period. If the strings feel lower than normal, if you can feel the rod, or if you can't feel any strings at all, I advise you to have the coil checked by a doctor or nurse – and use condoms in the meantime, because if it's incorrectly positioned, it will not work as a contraceptive.

While there don't appear to be any clear health advantages or disadvantages to using menstrual cups compared to using pads or tampons, there are clear economic and environmental advantages. It's been estimated that using a menstrual cup for 10 years would cost 5% of the price and produce 0.4% of the plastic waste than if you used 12 pads per period, or 7% of the cost and 6% of the plastic waste compared to 12 tampons per period.[18]

Pelvic organ prolapse

This means the descent of the pelvic organs (the uterus, bladder, bowel and vagina itself) into the vagina, due to weakening of the ligaments and muscles that hold the organs inside the pelvis. It is more common in women who have had babies, especially after vaginal births, but even having a Caesarean section does not protect you from a prolapse: all pregnancies put pressure on a woman's pelvic floor, no matter how the baby is born.

Other things that can increase the chance of prolapse are: increasing age, obesity, a chronic cough, constipation and menopause.

This can also happen after a hysterectomy, and in this case it's called vaginal vault prolapse. Symptoms include:

- A bulge or lump in the vagina (which can occasionally come out of the vagina).
- A dragging sensation in the pelvis.
- Backache.
- Difficulty emptying your bladder or bowel (e.g. needing to press on the bulge so you can pass urine or stool, needing to go more often than usual, feeling an unusual urgency or leaking urine).
- Difficulty having penetrative sex, discomfort or altered sensation.

If you are worried you should see your GP, who will take a full history and can perform an examination to determine whether there is indeed a prolapse.

Treatment for prolapse includes physiotherapy, vaginal oestrogen creams or tablets, use of vaginal pessaries, and in some cases surgery. It's also quite common to have a mild prolapse without any symptoms, in which case you don't need to do anything.

Tampons

Unlike menstrual cups, there are no concerns about using tampons with a coil. Tampons can be very convenient, although – as with cups – some women just don't like having to insert something into their vagina. Some women also find using tampons incredibly painful, such as if they have a very tight pelvic floor. There don't appear to be any health complications with tampon use, although, interestingly, one study has suggested that tampon use may protect against endometriosis.[19] (I think this finding is confounded by the fact that many of my patients with endometriosis don't use tampons because they find them too uncomfortable, which may be due to internal inflammation and scarring.)

Don't forget that tampons have a shelf life, so I recommend periodically replacing that 'emergency tampon' that most of us keep in the bottom of our handbag. Don't use a tampon if it has expired, the wrapper is torn, or if it got wet that time your coffee cup leaked all over your bag, etc.

Losing a tampon inside your vagina is also surprisingly common. I can't count the number of times that I've been called to remove a tampon during my career. While it often happens, I have never ever seen anyone with toxic shock syndrome (page 61), which is something that a lot of women worry about. It is exceedingly rare – but it's important to be aware of the signs.

Also, quite a lot of women who are sure they have lost a tampon inside are mistaken: they have either removed their tampon and forgotten about it, or it's fallen out while they've been on the toilet and they didn't notice. But that doesn't matter. It's best to check if you're concerned. And if it's not inside your vagina, I promise you it can't go any further up.

Pads

Pads are often overlooked due to the huge range of other products available. They're great because they're easy to keep in your bag 'just in case', they're good for when you're starting your periods and may not want to insert anything into your vagina, and they're good for lighter days when you don't want to wear a tampon. There is a wide range of options – with wings, without, thick, thin, cotton, organic, synthetic, reusable – so you can choose what suits you and your period. I advise you to avoid anything scented because the perfume can irritate the delicate vulval skin.

Period underwear

Period underwear has become incredibly popular over the last few years. Period pants look like normal underwear, but have an absorbent gusset with a moisture-wicking top layer to keep you feeling dry. These are a great choice for girls who have started their periods, as they can wear them to school without worrying about having to change them during the day (most brands recommend changing the pants after 12 hours).

Once you've worn them you rinse them then pop them in the wash as you would any other pair of pants, but usually without fabric softener, which can reduce their absorbency over time. I've been sent a vast array of period pants to try over the past few years, and I've been impressed by their quality, absorbency, and the fact that they generally feel very discreet. I think they're great for heavy days when you're worried that a tampon or cup might leak, or on lighter days towards the end of your period, but I know plenty of women who wear them throughout.

Toxic shock syndrome

Toxic shock syndrome (TSS) is an exceedingly rare condition, yet one that most people seem to have heard of. It seems to put some women off using tampons, due to the relation between TSS and their use. TSS is caused by a toxin, TSST-1, which is produced by *Staphylococcus aureus* bacteria, not by any kind of chemical that is in the tampon itself. If TSST-1 enters the bloodstream it causes a tremendous inflammatory reaction, resulting in an extremely high fever, vomiting, muscle aches and a skin rash. TSS can be life-threatening, and requires urgent medical attention. Thankfully it's exceedingly rare, with about 40 cases seen in the UK per year. About half of these cases are thought to be related to tampon use, and the remainder are usually associated with skin infections and burns.

Tampon use may be related to TSS because:

1. The collection of blood provides a perfect environment for bacteria to grow.
2. Inserting and removing tampons causes tiny micro-abrasions in the vaginal wall, allowing bacteria to enter the bloodstream. This sounds alarming, but vaginal penetration during sex or masturbation does the same thing.

Note that menstrual cups also collect blood inside your body. There have been a few cases of TSS reported with menstrual cup use.[20] Using organic tampons does not reduce the risk of TSS.

Given how rare TSS is, I don't think it's a reason to avoid tampons. My top tips to ensure safe tampon use are:

- Wash your hands before inserting a tampon.
- Don't leave a tampon in for more than 8 hours.
- Don't use a tampon that is too absorbent for your needs (e.g. don't use a super tampon for a relatively light flow because you're going out for the day and don't want to change your tampon).
- Don't use a tampon when you're not on your period.

Choosing to delay your period for a holiday or other occasion

Most of us have had that moment of dread: you look at your calendar, do some mental arithmetic, and realise that your period is going to arrive in the middle of a beach holiday. Don't you wish there was a way to prevent it!? Well, there are two possible methods, both of which involve the use of hormonal medications:

If you're on the combined oral contraceptive pill (COCP): The COCP is the type you take for 21 days then have a break for 4 or 7 days, during which you have a period. If you want to stop your period, you simply skip the 4- or 7-day break and start taking the next pack straight away. You won't have a bleed because you will maintain a constant hormone level. There are many more tailored ways of taking the COCP (see pages 240–2), but to delay one period for a holiday/event, this is how to do it.

If you use the progesterone-only pill (POP, the one with 28 of the same tablets in a pack), you cannot manipulate the timing of your period.

If you're not on the COCP: You can use Norethisterone, a synthetic progestogen tablet that you take three times per day, starting 3 days before your period is due and continuing for the duration of your trip/the time for which you want to stop your period. Your period will usually start about 2 or 3 days after stopping the tablets. It's important to be aware that Norethisterone can cause cramping, spotting, bloating, breast tenderness and mood swings, and your next period might be heavier than normal. Some women notice that the timing of their next period is also altered. This tablet can be prescribed by your GP or bought over the counter from some pharmacies: a pharmacist will ask you a series of questions relating to your health to ensure it's safe for you to take.

Please note that this method does not provide you with any form of contraception, so you still need to use another method at the same time (e.g. condoms), but you could use this method with a hormonal or a copper coil in place.

Speak to your GP/nurse/pharmacist for more info on this topic.

Since the timing of your period is related to hormonal changes in your body, there is no non-hormonal way to delay your period.

Chapter 3

How do I know if my periods are not normal?

Before we explore period problems, it's important to define what's *normal* first. As a general guide, a normal period:

- is predictable – you have some idea of when it's going arrive
- lasts less than a week
- is not too heavy
- is not too painful.

And you don't bleed in between periods.

This simple classification of a normal period allows for a huge spectrum of what's 'normal', but human beings are not a textbook and every woman will have a slightly different experience. If your period doesn't fit into this classification, don't panic. The information in the next few sections may help you decide whether you should go to your GP to seek help or discuss further investigations.

Now we will go on to discuss some periods that are not normal.

Irregular/absent periods

You should have a general idea of when your period is going to arrive. Many women report having an irregular cycle, but after further questioning they say that one month it was 28 days, the next 30 days, then 27 days. This is not an irregular cycle. While some people may have an extremely consistent length of cycle, it is normal for your cycle to vary by a few days each month.

A definition of an irregular menstrual cycle depends on how long it has been since your periods started. It is normal for periods to be irregular and haphazard for at least the first year after they start, because the hormonal cycle is still establishing itself.

The following are irregular menstrual cycles:

- A cycle length of less than 21 days or more than 45 days (between 1 and 3 years after your first ever period).
- A cycle length of less than 21 days or more than 35 days (3 years or more since your first ever period) *or* having under eight cycles per year.

Amenorrhoea is the term given to absent periods. It can be primary, which means your periods have never started (see page 43), or secondary, which means that you used to have normal periods but you haven't had one for at least 3 months.

Many factors – related to the normal functioning of your body (physiological), to your hormones (hormonal), or to the structure of your gynaecological organs (anatomical) – may cause irregular or absent periods after they have started, and these are listed below.

- Physiological, including:

Pregnancy – this is very quick and simple to exclude! A home urine pregnancy test is just as reliable as the ones in your GP's surgery or hospital.

Breastfeeding – this is called lactational amenorrhoea (see page 83).

- Hormonal, including:

Polycystic ovarian syndrome (PCOS; see page 125).

Hypothalamic amenorrhoea (page 148).

Thyroid disorders.

Hormone-secreting tumours such as prolactinomas, which are non-cancerous tumours in the pituitary gland in the brain. These secrete excess prolactin, and lead to a leakage of milk from your breasts in 80% of cases.

- Anatomical, including:

Cervical stenosis – this can occur after treatment to the cervix for precancerous cells. The cervix can become scarred shut, causing period blood to accumulate inside the uterus. During your period you may notice cramps or pain. The problem is relatively simple to fix with a small metal dilator, usually under general anaesthetic, to open up the cervix to drain the blood.

Asherman's syndrome – this is a build-up of scar tissue inside the uterus. It may develop after surgery inside the uterus, such as to terminate a pregnancy, treat a miscarriage or remove fibroids.

You may have one cycle that's a bit longer than is usual for you but then things go back to normal. This is often related to recent travel across time zones, a brief period of stress, such as an important deadline, or a recent illness. As long as your cycle goes back to normal there's nothing to worry about, and there's unlikely to be anything sinister going on.

Prolonged bleeding

The average length of a period is about 5 days: a period that lasts 9 days or more is classified as prolonged bleeding. This is more common during the first few years of having periods, and then as you move towards the menopause, because of erratic ovulation at each end of a woman's reproductive life. It can lead to anaemia if not treated (see page 70). Other causes are listed below.

- Hormonal, including:

Polycystic ovarian syndrome (PCOS; see page 125).

Thyroid disorders.

- Anatomical, including:

Adenomyosis (see page 107).

Fibroids.

Polyps.

Endometrial hyperplasia or cancer (see page 139).

Cervical cancer.

- Problems with a Caesarean scar.
- Infections.
- Blood-clotting disorders.
- Blood-thinning medications.
- The copper coil.

Anaemia

Anaemia means that you either have fewer red blood cells than normal, or the haemoglobin concentration in your red blood cells is low. There are several types of anaemia, with iron-deficiency anaemia being the type usually associated with heavy periods.

Iron deficiency is the most common micronutrient deficiency worldwide, and periods are the most common cause of this in women. In the UK 14% of non-pregnant women have iron-deficiency anaemia.[21]

Symptoms of anaemia

- Fatigue
- Shortness of breath
- Fainting
- Palpitations

- Headache
- Tinnitus
- Hair loss
- Restless leg syndrome
- Sore tongue
- Ulceration of the corners of the mouth (this is called 'angular stomatitis').

How severe your symptoms are can depend on how quickly the anaemia has developed. Someone who has had a slow, progressive decline in their haemoglobin level may be able to tolerate a shockingly low haemoglobin level much better than someone who had a sudden drop from an isolated heavy bleed. To put this into perspective, anaemia is defined as a haemoglobin level of less than 120g/l in a non-pregnant female: I'd estimate that most of my patients who are anaemic due to heavy periods have haemoglobin levels of 70–90g/l. The lowest I've ever seen was just under 29g/l. I was convinced the test result was wrong, as I couldn't believe that the patient was still standing with such a low level, but when I repeated her blood test myself and saw pale, watery blood running from her vein, I realised the test was indeed accurate.

Treatment usually involves iron tablet supplementation. It's advised that you take these with orange juice because vitamin C enhances absorption. You should avoid drinking tea and coffee within half an hour of taking iron tablets, because this can reduce absorption. A blood test should be repeated about 4 weeks after starting iron tablets to check how you're responding. Iron tablets can cause nausea, constipation and black stools, which makes them undesirable to some people, but if you're finding them difficult to tolerate, please see your doctor to discuss ways to combat this, as well as alternatives. It is possible to have an iron infusion, and if your haemoglobin is very low and you have a lot of symptoms it may be necessary to have a blood transfusion. Iron tablets should raise your haemoglobin by about 20g/l within 3–4 weeks; an iron infusion should do the same within one week. Each unit of blood should raise your level by 10g/l by the time it's finished transfusing.[22]

Identifying and treating the underlying cause of anaemia where possible is also important: this is why further investigations, such as an ultrasound scan, may be needed. While heavy periods are the most common cause of anaemia, it's important not to overlook non-gynaecological causes, such as bowel-related problems, simply because someone has a uterus!

Heavy periods

Medical textbooks tend to define a heavy period as a total blood loss of 80ml or more, but that's not very easy to check and I feel that this number is meaningless. Passing large blood clots, needing to change your pad or tampon at least every hour for several hours in a row (or a menstrual cup at least every 4 hours) or wearing a pad and tampon/cup together are also signs that your bleeding is quite heavy. However, we are all different, so my preferred description of a heavy period comes from the National Institute for Health and Care Excellence (NICE) website*: 'Any excessive menstrual blood loss which interferes with a woman's physical, emotional, social and material quality of life, and which can occur alone or in combination with other symptoms.'

It's estimated that 3.5 million women in the UK experience heavy periods, but about half have never sought medical advice for this treatable condition. Heavy periods can have a huge impact on your quality of life, and the things that you're able to do. It's estimated that 5.5 million work days are lost per year due to heavy periods, but this doesn't begin to provide any insight into the number of social occasions, exercise sessions and date nights lost, or the mundane, yet essential, activities that become more difficult or impossible due to heavy periods. Heavy periods can also disrupt sleep, with many women reporting that they have to get up several times in a night to change their period products, pyjamas or sheets, which has a huge knock-on effect on how they func-

* NICE (the National Institute for Health and Care Excellence) is the organisation responsible for promoting the provision of optimal healthcare for patients through the development of evidence-based guidelines, appraising new treatments and technologies, and promoting change towards best practice. https://www.nice.org.uk/guidance/ng88/chapter/Context

tion the following day. Heavy bleeding can be scary: it's not unusual to see a woman in A&E reporting heavy bleeding that requires urgent treatment, which may include a blood transfusion. Not every woman with heavy periods will need a blood transfusion, but heavy periods are a very common cause of anaemia, which can usually be treated with iron tablets, making women feel a lot more energetic and generally better. Anaemia is covered in more depth on pages 70–72.

In about 50% of cases, no cause is found to explain heavy periods, but medications such as tranexamic acid, mefenamic acid and hormonal contraception can still help in these cases. Surgery such as endometrial ablation and hysterectomy can also be used if medical treatment is unsuccessful. Other causes are listed below.

- Hormonal, including:

Polycystic ovarian syndrome (PCOS).

Thyroid disorders.

Perimenopause.

- Anatomical, including:

Adenomyosis.

Fibroids.

Polyps.

Endometrial hyperplasia or cancer.

Cervical cancer.

Blood-clotting disorders.

Blood-thinning medications.

The copper coil.

Light periods

While heavy periods tend to attract more attention, there are lots of women who have quite light periods where they barely need to wear a pad or a tampon, or their period just lasts a day or two. If your period is generally very light, there is nothing to worry about – this is normal for some women, and there is no association with light periods and problems getting pregnant in the future. However, if your period changes and suddenly becomes light, and this lasts more than two or three cycles, or if you have other symptoms that are concerning you, you should consider discussing this with your doctor.

Causes of light periods

- Thyroid problems.
- Sudden or significant weight loss.
- Excessive exercise.

- Stress or anxiety.
- Recent travel across time zones.
- Perimenopause.
- PCOS (periods are typically heavier, but light periods are also possible).
- Implantation bleeding (the bleeding you may get when a fertilised egg starts to burrow itself into the endometrium early on in pregnancy. Many women understandably mistake this for a period, as they don't realise they're pregnant. A pregnancy test would still be negative at this stage).
- Taking the contraceptive pill, or using the implant, injection or hormonal coil (this is related to their ability to keep the endometrium thin, which is part of the way they work).

Painful periods

Also known as **dysmenorrhoea**, painful periods may be classified as primary (where no obvious cause is found) or secondary (occurring as a result of an identifiable cause – see list on page 78). Patients often tell me, 'I have a really high pain threshold', which always worries me, because I wonder what kind of awful pain they've been putting up with at home. A small amount of pain just before and during your period is normal, but pain shouldn't be excessive: it should not disrupt your normal activities or require more than the occasional paracetamol or ibuprofen tablet. Taking over-the-counter painkillers isn't going to mask anything sinister, but you certainly shouldn't be clock-watching or having to set a timer on your phone to tell you when you can take your next dose. You may also experience nausea, vomiting, diarrhoea, sweating, heart palpitations or fainting. If you regularly have any of these symptoms, you should seek medical attention.

Period pain happens when the endometrium produces prostaglandins. These cause the rhythmic contraction of the uterus, the constriction of blood vessels, and a lack of blood supply to the uterus, which results in the cramping pain that most women know all too well. With women who suffer from severe period pain, it has been shown that they produce too much of these prostaglandins, and higher levels correlate directly with higher levels of pain.[23] They may also have stronger uterine muscle contractions, which results in a greater reduction in the blood supply and, ultimately, oxygen supply, to the uterine muscle when it's contracting, which also contributes to the pain. This is often described as being like a heart attack in your uterus, because what's going on from a biological perspective is similar. Even when no underlying condition can be found to explain your period pain, there really is something going on at a cellular and chemical level – you're not imagining it. You may feel pain in your lower abdomen and back, and this may travel down your thighs – this is due to cross-communication between the nerves in your pelvis.

Period pain can have a negative impact on your quality of life and interfere with the daily activities you need and want to do. It also frequently disrupts sleep: many people report that their pain is worse at night, which may be due to the fact that we're less distracted by other things, so the pain gets more of our attention. Many people say that lying in the foetal position (i.e. on their side, curled up in a ball) helps – perhaps because it relaxes your abdominal muscles, which may be contributing to pain.

Pain that relates to an underlying condition can often last longer than your period, and is often associated with other symptoms such as heavy or prolonged bleeding. That's why the lists of symptoms here are quite repetitive. They include:

- Hormonal, including:

Polycystic ovarian syndrome (PCOS).

Perimenopause.

- Anatomical, including:

Endometriosis.

Adenomyosis.

Fibroids.

Polyps.

Endometrial hyperplasia or cancer.

Cervical cancer.

- The copper coil.
- Pelvic inflammatory disease.

Unscheduled bleeding

This means any vaginal bleeding when you're not having your period. Doctors split this into two distinct types of bleeding:

- Intermenstrual bleeding (IMB) – any vaginal bleeding between periods.
- Postcoital bleeding (PCB) – bleeding after sex.

While these symptoms are quite common, with IMB occurring in about 17% of women and PCB in 6%,[24] they can be quite alarming because they may be a symptom of gynaecological cancer, and therefore it is important that you speak to your GP about them. Thankfully in most cases it's not cancer, but your doctor will want to be sure of this, as well as try to relieve your symptoms where possible.

Cervical cancer is the diagnosis that everyone worries about. The chance of this is low, but it does need to be ruled out.

This is done by examining your cervix during a speculum examination – the first step in investigating unscheduled bleeding. If something looks abnormal, you will be referred to the colposcopy clinic, where we will do an in-depth examination of your cervix using a microscope. We can also take a biopsy of any unusual areas that need further assessment.

Up to 40% of women who are eventually diagnosed with cervical cancer have bleeding after sex. However, the chance of having cervical cancer if you have bleeding after sex is very low: it's 1 in 44,000 if you're aged 20–24 and increases with age up to 1 in 2,400 if you're 45–54.[25] If you have unscheduled bleeding and have had a recent smear test that was normal, you should still see your doctor. While the chance of cervical cancer being missed in a smear test is low, it's not zero, and a smear test doesn't check for any other abnormalities, cancerous or otherwise, that could be the reason for your bleeding. If you haven't had one recently, then you can have one done at the same time as the examination of your cervix, but if the nurse sees anything abnormal on your cervix while they are doing the examination, you will still need to go to the colposcopy clinic.

Endometrial cancer or hyperplasia (precancerous cells) can also result in bleeding. Abnormalities on an ultrasound scan may suggest the presence of these conditions, and these can be diagnosed by taking a biopsy from the endometrial lining. Endometrial cancer is rare before the menopause: it's estimated that the chance of having endometrial cancer if you have bleeding between your periods is 0.5%.[26]

Vulval and vaginal cancers are very rare, but can also present with this type of bleeding, so we will always examine your vulva and vagina as part of our investigations.

In most cases the bleeding has a benign (non-cancerous) cause. These include:

- Cervical ectropion (see pages 14–16).
- Causes related to contraception – bleeding is common when starting progesterone-only methods, including POP and the hormonal coil, or with COCPs that contain lower doses of oestrogen (e.g. 20 micrograms vs 35 micrograms ethinyestradiol, a synthetic oestrogen commonly found in COCPs).
- Infections.
- Endometrial or cervical polyps.
- Fibroids.
- Ovulation bleeding.
- Pregnancy (e.g. implantation bleeding, miscarriage, ectopic pregnancy).
- Chronic skin conditions, including lichen sclerosus (see box below).
- Atrophic changes to the vulval and vaginal tissues. This means that the tissues become thin and inflamed. This is usually related to low oestrogen during menopause, but this can also occur when breastfeeding.

The first four causes are the most common.

Lichen sclerosus

Lichen sclerosus (LS) is a chronic inflammatory skin condition that affects 1 in 70 people and typically involves the skin of the vulva and anus. It is most common in the over-50s, but can arise at any age, including during childhood. It is not an infection, cannot be spread from person to person, and has nothing to do with sexual contact.

Symptoms:

- Itching.
- Changes in appearance of the vulva, including narrowing of vaginal opening, shrinkage of the labia minora, general tightening and thinning of the skin.
- White patches (loss of skin pigmentation).
- Darker patches (hyperpigmentation) can also develop over time.
- Fissures (small cuts in the skin).
- Generalised pain and discomfort that is often worse with friction, during sex and when opening bowels.

Unfortunately, lichen sclerosus is often misdiagnosed as thrush/a yeast infection. While some of the symptoms may be similar, thrush treatments will not work for LS. Using over-the-counter vulval washes and wipes will not help either; instead, they are likely to make the skin more irritated and inflamed. A small biopsy may be required to confirm the diagnosis, because there are several other skin conditions that can affect the vulva that need to be ruled out. Steroid ointment (e.g. Clobetasol) and calcineurin inhibitors (e.g. Tacrolimus) are the most common treatments. Not only do they reduce symptoms, but they can also reduce the risk of a woman developing vulval cancer, which is a complication of lichen sclerosus that may affect about 4% of women with this condition.

Lactational amenorrhoea

This means that your periods have stopped due to breastfeeding. It happens because when a baby suckles at your breast, this stops the usual communication loop between the brain and the ovary. As a result, your periods will stop.

Breastfeeding can be used as a form of contraception ONLY if you meet the following three criteria, as defined by the Faculty of Sexual and Reproductive Health:[27]

- Your baby is under 6 months old.
- You are exclusively breastfeeding (that is, breastfeeding at least every 4 hours during the day, and every 6 hours at night).
- You are not having periods.

Note: Pumping breast milk may make this method less effective due to the baby spending less time at the breast and less suckling stimulation, which might allow the usual brain–ovary communication to resume.

The failure rate of this contraceptive method is about 1–2%, which means if 100 breastfeeding mothers used this method of contraception, 1 or 2 would unintentionally get pregnant. If at any point, even within the first six months, all three of these criteria do not apply, you must use an alternative form of contraception if you do not want to get pregnant. There are plenty of forms of contraception that you can safely use while breastfeeding: you can discuss contraception with a midwife on the postnatal ward or with your GP at your postnatal check.

'When will my periods start again after having my baby?' is a very good question, and one that's difficult to answer. Many women find that their periods return as their baby starts to drop night feeds, and also as the length of time between daytime feeds increases. Some women have the opposite experience: they stop breastfeeding completely and find that their period doesn't return for several months.

Speak to your GP if your periods haven't come back 3 months after stopping breastfeeding entirely.

Chapter 4

Which conditions can cause problems with periods?

A wide range of conditions can cause problems with periods, and I have summarised many of these here. Some are very common, some less so, and some you might never have heard of. However, I have noticed in conversations with patients that many women don't know about even some of the more common conditions because we are just not taught about them. There is also so much misinformation online about gynaecological health, so I'm on a mission, along with some excellent colleagues, to stamp this out – while providing you with high-quality, reliable facts and information.

Just because you have symptoms of a particular condition, this doesn't mean that you definitely have it. Patients often tell me they delayed seeking help because they weren't sure what was wrong with them. Please remember that it's not your responsibility to diagnose yourself before seeing a doctor.

If you think you may have a certain condition, or you're worried about something, please let your doctor know. It's helpful for us to consider that potential diagnosis, and if you don't have that condition, then we can reassure you and tell you why we don't think you have it.

Endometriosis

Endometriosis is the presence of endometrium-like tissue outside the uterus. It affects about 10% of women. Endometrial-like tissue can grow on the peritoneum, which is the membrane-like tissue that lines the inside of the abdomen, pelvic cavity and all the organs including the bladder and bowel, as well as on the ovaries. In about 10% of cases it also grows in the chest, where it can cause chest pain and lead to coughing up blood. Wherever endometrial-like tissue is present, it grows in response to oestrogen. This tissue is able to produce its own oestrogen, independent of the ovaries, along with other chemicals responsible for pain and inflammation. So how does this tissue get there? Does it travel there and seed itself? Or was it always there, and just starts to become active and grow once you start having your periods? No one is entirely sure, but I want to reassure you that there is a great deal of research being done to try to understand this condition better, to improve diagnosis and treatment. It's a myth that a woman can be 'too young to have endometriosis': a review of surgical studies showed that in adolescents with symptoms suggestive of endometriosis, 64% did indeed have the disease, confirmed by diagnostic laparoscopy.[28]

There are different type of endometriosis:

Superficial or peritoneal endometriosis – This means the endometrial-like tissue grows on the surface of the peritoneum, including the surface of pelvic organs. It is usually present in small plaques that are only a few millimetres deep. In their early stages they can look like very small clear, white, pink or red bubbles or patches on the surface. Later they become a darker brown, blue or black, and can cause some puckering of the surface of the peritoneum.

Deep endometriosis or deep infiltrating endometriosis – This is when the endometriosis invades deeply into pelvic structures such as the bladder, bowel or ligaments. Rectovaginal endometriosis is the most severe form of this: involving significant scarring between the rectum and vagina due to endometriosis causing the organs to become completely stuck together, rather than being able to glide gently over one another.

Ovarian endometriosis – This means the presence of an endometrioma on the ovary, which is an endometriosis-containing cyst. These are also called 'chocolate cysts' (see page 21). About two-thirds of people with endometriomas will also have deep endometriosis.

Endometriosis is not the same thing as endometritis, which is the inflammation of the lining of the uterus – this condition can occur after birth or a surgical procedure on the uterus.

One of the problems with endometriosis is the lack of awareness of this condition and how detrimental it can be to women's health and livelihoods. In England, the average time it takes to get diagnosed is 7 to 9 years, which is far too long. Data collected from 10,000 women with endometriosis in England show that 58% visited the GP at least ten times before being diagnosed, 43% went to hospital at least five times, and 53% went to A&E before being diagnosed.[29] This is devastating to read, but clearly much more devastating to experience this. Since the symptoms of endometriosis are not always gynae-specific (see below), many women see multiple other doctors before seeing a gynaecologist, which is why all doctors and healthcare professionals need to be educated about endometriosis. While I learned very little about it in medical school, today this is changing. I am incredibly grateful to my patients with endometriosis, and the countless women who share their very raw, personal stories online, because they have educated me about what it means to live with endometriosis; a textbook can only tell you so much. I'm so sorry for everyone who has not been heard and whose stories have been dismissed.

I recently did a webinar with Carla Cressy, founder and CEO of the Endometriosis Foundation. Carla has had eight operations relating to endometriosis, including the removal of her uterus, fallopian tubes and ovaries and a bowel resection with a stoma that has since been reversed. One member of the audience asked Carla how to get doctors to take their symptoms more seriously, and her best advice was to read the NICE guidelines for diagnosing endometriosis – or even print them out to take with you to your consultation. These are evidence-based guidelines that set out a standard of care for women with suspected and confirmed endometriosis. The information that follows about diagnosis and management of endometriosis is based on these guidelines.[30]

I'm often asked whether having endometriosis increases your risk of cancer. The answer is: *very* slightly. Large population studies show higher rates of ovarian, breast and thyroid cancer in women with endometriosis, but Table 4.1 shows that the absolute increase in number of cases compared to the general population is small.[31]

	General population	People with endometriosis	Increased risk with endo
Ovarian cancer	1.3%	2.5%	1.2%
Breast cancer	12.8%	13.3%	0.5%
Thyroid cancer	1.3%	1.8%	0.5%

Table 4.1. *The risk of ovarian, breast and thyroid cancers associated with endometriosis compared to the risk in the general population.*

There are no known ways in which these risks can be reduced, but it remains important for women with endometriosis to attend breast screening and to ensure they maintain a healthy lifestyle.

Symptoms of endometriosis

Endometriosis is the most common cause of secondary dysmenorrhoea, which means painful periods with an identifiable cause. While painful periods may be a symptom of endometriosis, there are many more symptoms, including:

- Abdominal / pelvic pain.
- Heavy periods – not a prerequisite for endometriosis, and can be suggestive of adenomyosis, which is commonly found with endometriosis (see pages 107–14).
- Pain during sex.
- Pain when opening bowels (pooing) or blood in the stool around the time of your period.
- Pain on passing urine (weeing) or blood in your urine around the time of your period.
- Fertility problems – 50% of women experiencing fertility problems are known, or subsequently found, to have endometriosis (see pages 105–7).
- Cyclical swelling and pain in a scar (e.g. a C-section scar or laparoscopy scar). This means pain and swelling in a scar that contains endometriosis. It usually worsens around the time of your period.
- Mental health problems.
- Fatigue.

As you can see, the symptoms are quite varied and don't all point directly to a gynae problem. I vividly remember a patient with endometriosis I met in A&E. I was down there one evening seeing a few patients who had been referred to the gynae team and I got chatting to one of the general surgery doctors – mainly because I'd had a really stressful day and wanted a bit of a chat, but also because I'm always intrigued by what other teams are up to. He mentioned that he had seen a woman in her twenties with a recurrent infection in her belly button, about a year after having her appendix removed via keyhole surgery. He wasn't sure what to do about it because, despite the woman taking antibiotics, it always came back, and none of the swabs they'd taken grew any unusual types of bacteria to suggest a more appropriate antibiotic. He also mentioned that he felt sorry for her, having to come to the hospital every month or so . . .

That made me sit up and take notice. 'Every month or so, you say? Can I have a look?' I asked.

He looked perplexed, but said, 'Be my guest!'

The patient was lovely, and was delighted to show me her gunky belly button if it meant a possible solution. On seeing it, I immediately suspected endometriosis. After speaking to her for about five minutes, I'd found out that she had classic symptoms of endometriosis which had flared up about 2 years before, after she'd stopped taking the contraceptive pill, because she'd read scary things about its side effects online. After multiple trips to her GP and A&E she had ended up having her appendix removed for suspected appendicitis, although the lab analysis of her appendix came back normal. The two small surgical cuts on her abdomen had healed nicely, but the belly button cut just refused to heal. After further questioning, she mentioned that it produced a mucky-looking, blood-stained discharge . . . when she had her period! Diagnosis made – endometriosis in the belly button scar. I took her details and arranged for her to be seen in the gynaecology clinic. She had the scar refashioned to remove the endometriosis to stop the recurrent bleeding and she restarted the pill to help reduce her pelvic pain. Admittedly, it's not the most common way for endometriosis to be diagnosed, but it goes to show that endometriosis doesn't always present with 'bad periods'. Giving someone the opportunity to tell their full story, with a few targeted questions, can get you to the correct diagnosis.

Keeping a diary of symptoms can be very helpful when it comes to describing your symptoms to your doctor. You can do this using your phone calendar, a period-tracking app or good old-fashioned pen and paper. It should include information about the symptoms you're experiencing and your menstrual cycle.

Given the types of symptoms associated with endometriosis, and how severe they can be, it's unsurprising that they can have a significant negative impact on your daily life. In a survey carried out by the BBC of over 13,500 women with endometriosis, most said it had negatively affected their education, career and sex life. Nearly all women also said it had affected their mental health: around half had experienced suicidal thoughts as a result.[32]

After the menopause, with the dramatic drop in oestrogen levels, endometriosis will be far less active and symptoms tend to abate. A small number of women will continue to have symptoms. This may be related to the tissue's ability to make its own oestrogen, or to using HRT, particularly oestrogen-only HRT, which can cause endometriosis to flare up in some cases. However, it doesn't rule out the use of HRT for menopausal symptoms. Your doctor will be able to discuss suitable options for you.

Diagnosis of endometriosis

Examination of your abdomen is a useful first step in making a diagnosis. This may include feeling your abdomen from above, and an internal examination. This allows us to understand where exactly the pain is, and feel for any lumps and masses. During an internal examination we may feel thickened uterosacral nodules at the back of the uterus, which are classic symptoms of deep endometriosis, or we may feel that your uterus doesn't move very much upon manipulation, which can be a sign of endometriosis-related scarring. It's also important to rule out any other conditions because the symptoms of endometriosis overlap with those of many other gynaecological and non-gynaecological conditions. For many people with endometriosis, however, the results of this examination may be entirely normal.

An ultrasound scan is usually the first investigation to be offered, but it has its limitations. Pelvic ultrasounds should ideally be performed internally, using a probe that is inserted into the vagina. Ovarian endometriosis can be diagnosed relatively easily on an ultrasound scan. Sometimes a woman's ovaries are described as 'kissing ovaries', which means they sit behind your uterus and are pulled together: it is endometriosis scar tissue that pulls them into this abnormal positioning, suggesting the presence of deep endometriosis. In the absence of kissing ovaries, deep endometriosis can otherwise be picked up on an ultrasound scan when this is done by someone who is particularly experienced in diagnosing endometriosis. Superficial endometriosis is incredibly difficult to detect using ultrasound scanning, even when done by an expert, because the deposits are tiny – so if you have symptoms suggestive of endometriosis but your scan is normal that does not mean that you do not have endometriosis.

Before surgery, magnetic resonance imaging (MRI) scanning can be useful to provide your surgeon with further information about where the disease is and which organs may be stuck together. But it is not very useful for diagnosing superficial endometriosis, and therefore it isn't generally used for diagnosis. Unfortunately, many women who are suffering pain are told, 'Your scan is normal so there's nothing wrong with you', which completely invalidates their experience. Your scan may be normal, but you still have pain, which is very real. If your ultrasound scan is normal, the next step is to consider either a diagnostic laparoscopy or a trial of hormonal treatment.

Diagnostic laparoscopy is keyhole surgery to look inside your abdomen and pelvis for endometriosis. The surgery is explained on page 275. It involves looking at your uterus, fallopian tubes, ovaries, the peritoneal surfaces of your abdomen and pelvis and your diaphragm, which is another place where endometriosis may be found. Small biopsies may be taken that can be examined under a microscope to confirm the diagnosis of endometriosis. If you're trying to get pregnant, your surgeon may suggest doing a 'dye test' at the same time to check that your fallopian tubes are open. Overall, laparoscopy is a safe procedure, but it does carry some risks, which include damage to blood vessels and pelvic organs, such as the bladder and bowel. This is one of the reasons that there is an increasing tendency to offer a trial of hormonal treatment before proceeding to surgery, because if the medication resolves your pain, you can avoid the potential risks associated with surgery. The European guidelines on endometriosis produced by the European Society of Human Reproduction and Embryology (ESHRE; see reference 31) were recently updated to state that diagnostic laparoscopy should only be used where scans are normal and a trial of hormonal treatment has been ineffective,[31] and it is likely that the NICE guidelines will shortly be updated to state the same. Of course, you and your gynaecologist should discuss what is most appropriate for your individual case. Many women have told me they felt forced to take hormonal treatments, but you should never feel pressurised to accept or undergo any form of medical treatment or intervention.

I believe that the rationale for using hormones is often poorly explained, so I've attempted to do just that in the section below (and later on in the longer section on hormonal treatments; see page 233).

There are currently no blood tests that can be used to confirm or rule out a diagnosis of endometriosis. CA-125 is a tumour marker that can be checked on a blood test, and it's often used to help diagnose ovarian cancer. CA-125 is often raised in women with endometriosis, but the test can also be normal in women with endometriosis. Since CA-125 is also raised by many other conditions, this is not accurate enough to be used to help diagnose endometriosis.

Treatment options for endometriosis

Pregnancy is *not* a treatment for endometriosis. Unfortunately, I've heard this suggested far too often. Not only is it factually incorrect, but it's also a hurtful, dismissive suggestion to make. Your endometriosis is unlikely to cause you significant pain during pregnancy, but it will still be there after your baby is born.

Non-hormonal treatments

NSAIDs (non-steroidal anti-inflammatory drugs) such as naproxen and ibuprofen – These may help to a degree, and you can try them yourself at home, but they are low down on the list of effective treatments.

Tranexamic acid – This drug helps with heavy periods by reducing blood loss. Anecdotally, some patients with endometriosis have found that it reduces their period pain, but there is no evidence to suggest that it does anything to the endometriosis itself.

Pelvic floor physiotherapy – This might not be exactly what springs to mind when thinking about endometriosis, and while there isn't a great deal of published data on how effective it is, a lot of patients report relief when using pelvic floor physiotherapy. When you experience chronic pain, you can often hold tension in the muscles, and it is not uncommon to find excessively tight pelvic floor muscles in women with endometriosis. The pelvic floor isn't designed to be under constant tension, so this results in pain. Physiotherapists can help with muscle relaxation, stretching and mobilisation techniques to relieve this tightness and pain.

Psychological support – 95% of the 10,000 women who responded to the APPG Endometriosis survey reported that their endometriosis had negatively affected their wellbeing; 90% said they would have liked access to psychological therapies, but this was not offered.[29] Many endometriosis teams are able to offer access to this, but you can also ask your GP for a referral to the NHS Talking Therapies service.

Hormonal treatments

Hormonal medications are used to reduce endometriosis symptoms, based on the principle that endometriosis relies on oestrogen to function, which causes pain, inflammation and ultimately scarring. These medications aim to keep the endometriosis deposits thin and relatively inactive. While these meds aren't going to make the endometriosis go away entirely, studies consistently show that they can reduce the severity of symptoms and improve quality of life. The downside of hormonal medications is the side effects, which many people find intolerable, but there is no way of knowing whether you're going to have a positive or negative experience without trying them. These medications are not suitable for women who want to get pregnant, but they have no long-term impact on your fertility.

Combined oral contraceptive pill (COCP) – While these do contain oestrogen, it's the progesterone component that works to suppress endometriotic lesions. The COCP can reduce period pain, non-cyclical pelvic pain (i.e. pelvic pain when you're not having your period), pain during sex, and pain with bowel movements. Studies comparing ultrasound evidence of endometriosis before and after 12 months of COCP use have shown that it can reduce the size of endometriomas and disease on the uterosacral ligaments (which attach the uterus to the back of the pelvic bone).[33] The COCP is commonly prescribed after endometriosis surgery to reduce the recurrence of symptoms, and has been shown to reduce the chance of endometriomas recurring after removal.[34] There is no clear evidence that one type of pill is better than another, but taking it continuously without the pill-free week may be most effective.[35] The combined contraceptive ring and patch are also effective alternatives.

Progesterone-only contraceptives – The progestogen-only pill, implant and injection have similarly been shown to reduce pain symptoms, with up to two-thirds of women reporting an improvement.[36] They are useful if you cannot take the COCP, but do not offer such predictable bleeding patterns.

Hormonal coil – This is a popular method of reducing pain symptoms.[37] Its benefit is that once it's there you can forget about it so you don't need to take a tablet every day. Levonorgestrel, its active ingredient, can be found within the peritoneal fluid (peritoneal fluid is fluid inside the abdominal and pelvic cavity), which is thought to be how the coil reduces the pain associated with peritoneal endometriosis deposits.[38] It can also be used to reduce the recurrence of pain symptoms after surgery, and when used over the long term after surgery the hormonal coil appears to be as effective as the COCP.[39] The hormonal coil is licensed for use as a contraceptive for up to 6 years, but many women report that its pain-reducing effect wears off earlier than this.

GnRH (gonadotrophin-releasing hormone) analogues – These induce a temporary menopause: 90% of women will stop having periods entirely. They are highly effective at reducing endometriosis pain, but they cause menopausal side effects. They should not be used for longer than 6 months without using 'add-back' HRT, the use of HRT to reduce menopausal symptoms and provide bone protection, but doesn't reduce their pain-reducing effects. It is unusual to use them over the long term, but they are often used for a few months before surgery, with the aim of reducing the blood supply to endometriosis lesions intended for removal, reducing adhesions (internal scar tissue) and overall inflammation. They can also be used for a short period after surgery to reduce the risk of disease recurrence.

Surgical treatments

Surgery can play a role in diagnosis and treatment. Some endometriosis operations can be performed by general gynaecologists, but complex surgery needs to be carried out by a gynaecologist who has specialist training in endometriosis surgery (as explained on pages 278–9).

Diagnostic laparoscopy – This is keyhole surgery to investigate pelvic pain, or abnormalities seen on a scan, which often turns out to be endometriosis. In some cases, the endometriosis may be treated during the same operation. In many cases it isn't, and it can be frustrating and disappointing to wake up from an operation to hear that you have endometriosis but that your surgeon hasn't done anything to remove it. This doesn't mean they are a bad surgeon, though – quite the opposite, in fact, because a good surgeon is someone who knows when *not* to operate. While general gynaecologists can be very good at diagnosing endometriosis during laparoscopy, if it is severe it needs to be removed by someone with specialist training in endometriosis excision, supported by other specialist surgeons as necessary.

Excisional surgery – Surgery for endometriosis increasingly involves excision (cutting out) of endometriosis rather than ablation (destroying the endometriosis using techniques such as burning or laser), because this is likely to be more effective at reducing pain.[40] Up to 30% of women who undergo excisional surgery will experience recurrence or worsening of their pain within 3 years of surgery, and this increases to 50% in 5 years.[41] Hormonal medications are offered after surgery to reduce the risk of symptom and disease recurrence, as discussed above.

Hysterectomy – This is not a cure for endometriosis but may be appropriate in some situations, particularly if you have adenomyosis, which often co-exists with endometriosis. Removing the uterus will make your periods stop, but remember that endometriosis isn't about what's going on inside the uterus; it's about the presence of endometriosis deposits outside, so these all need to be removed at the same time as your uterus. Many surgeons recommend removal of the ovaries at the same time, because otherwise the ongoing oestrogen production by the ovaries could result in further growth of any endometriosis that was not removed at the time of the hysterectomy, but each case is individual. Removal of your ovaries will result in surgical menopause (see pages 283–4).

Endometriosis centres

In 2003 a group of gynaecologists from the UK acknowledged that there was a need to improve the quality and consistency of surgical treatment for women with endometriosis. This led to the establishment of specialist endometriosis centres, accredited by the British Society of Gynaecological Endoscopy (BSGE). These aim to reduce the variation in treatment provided, ensure high-quality surgery by specialists with the appropriate surgical expertise, and reduce waiting times, while monitoring patient outcomes. There are 63 centres in the UK, and each has its accreditation reviewed annually.

The BSGE has stated that the following are necessary for a hospital to become – and maintain its status as – an endometriosis centre:

- **A named gynaecologist**: This is someone who has had specialist training in advanced laparoscopic surgery and treatment of endometriosis, and runs a specialist endometriosis clinic. Excision of recto-vaginal endometriosis (that is, deep endometriosis in between the uterus and bowel) is one of the most complicated procedures that specialist endometriosis surgeons need to be competent to perform, and the BSGE states that each named endometriosis surgeon must perform at least 12 operations of this type annually to maintain their skills. Each surgeon must also submit a video of one of these complex operations, to be reviewed by the BSGE. These videos are recorded via the laparoscopic camera.
- **A supporting surgeon**: This is a colorectal surgeon who is involved with operations where endometriosis affects the bowel and where a bowel resection (removing a section of bowel) or formation of a stoma (when the end of the bowel is brought out onto the abdomen to divert stool into a bag) may be required. This may also include a urologist, who would be involved if endometriosis is affecting the bladder or ureter (the tube that transports urine from the kidney to the bladder). Other named specialists may also be involved, including pain specialists, radiologists, fertility specialists and physiotherapists.

- **A specialist endometriosis nurse**: These nurses are invaluable! They provide advice and support to patients throughout their journey – for example, with logistics related to their treatment or signposting other sources of support, such as peer-led groups. They usually give patients their telephone number or email address so they can act as a direct line of contact between the patient and the rest of the team.
- **Data collection**: A database of patients with severe endometriosis treated by the team must be kept for review. These patients must be followed up for at least 2 years.

When should I be referred to an endometriosis centre?

The criteria for referral to an endometriosis centre are confirmed or suspected endometriosis that involves:

- the bladder, bowel or ureter
- anywhere outside the pelvis – most commonly, the chest.

Your GP or a general gynaecologist can make the referral.

Endometriosis and fertility

If you google endometriosis and fertility, you're likely to come away thinking it's impossible to get pregnant if you have endometriosis. This is not true. However, we do see higher rates of fertility problems if you have endometriosis: between 30% and 50% of women with endometriosis have trouble conceiving, compared to 15% of the general population.

There are a few ways in which endometriosis may make it more challenging to get pregnant. These include:

- Damage to the ovaries as a result of endometriosis surgery or the disease itself.
- Blockage of the fallopian tubes, or impaired movement of the tubes as a result of surrounding endometriosis scarring. (It might surprise you to know that, in order to function normally, the fallopian tubes have to be free and mobile to move around in the pelvis to pick up eggs and to transport them into the uterus. They can be blocked inside, or they may be surrounded by scarring from the outside that stops them from moving in their normal way.
- An endometrium that is less receptive to implantation.

- Co-existence of adenomyosis, which is similarly known to negatively impact fertility.
- Painful sex, leading to reduced frequency of sex.

While hormonal treatments are commonly used to reduce endometriosis symptoms, they do not damage your fertility in the long term – in fact, there is some evidence to suggest that women who used this after surgery had a higher chance of pregnancy later, when they tried to conceive, compared to women who didn't use anything after surgery.[31]

Surgery to treat superficial/peritoneal endometriosis has been shown to improve pregnancy rates if you have already been trying to get pregnant without success for both spontaneous conception and IVF pregnancies.[42,43] There is less clear evidence to prove that surgery for deep endometriosis improves pregnancy rates, and as such must be considered on an individual basis because it may not be the right thing to undertake a potentially complex operation with a risk of serious complications, if we cannot be sure that it will increase the chance of a successful pregnancy. Further studies into this are ongoing. Excision of endometriomas greater than 4cm in size may improve the rate of spontaneous pregnancy, and removal of those greater than 3cm can be considered prior to IVF if it is felt it could improve access to the eggs during retrieval and may subsequently improve pregnancy rates.[31]

The Endometriosis Fertility Index (EFI) can be useful to predict your personalised chance of getting pregnant spontaneously after surgery based on your age, previous pregnancy history and findings at the time of surgery.

Most women with endometriosis do go on to get pregnant and will have successful pregnancies. There may be a higher chance of needing a Caesarean section during labour if you have endometriosis, but that does not mean that you cannot try for a vaginal birth if you wish to.

I've said it before, but I'll say it again . . . pregnancy does not cure endometriosis. And please do use contraception if you have endometriosis and don't want to get pregnant just yet.

Adenomyosis

Adenomyosis is a condition in which endometrial-like tissue invades the muscle layer, as shown in Figure 4.1. Even though it's in the wrong place, it still responds to your hormones throughout your menstrual cycle, so it thickens up and sheds. However, it gets trapped, resulting in painful periods, and over time it results in thickening and scarring of the muscle layer, causing the uterus to become enlarged and often more rounded in shape. This change in the configuration of the muscle is also thought to contribute to heavy periods, which are a common feature of adenomyosis, because the muscle is unable to contract as it usually would to stop bleeding.

Adenomyosis is often referred to as 'endometriosis of the uterus', which makes sense but can be confusing. Essentially, in both conditions there's endometrial-like tissue in the wrong place, but with endometriosis that tissue is *outside* the uterus, whereas with adenomyosis it's *inside* the uterus. We don't really understand how or why adenomyosis occurs, but we do know that if a woman has adenomyosis she has a 70% chance of having endometriosis too, and a 50% chance of having fibroids.[44] Adenomyosis is also more common if you are over 30 or have had a baby.

Adenomyosis has been very under-represented and under-researched, and very few patients I speak to have ever heard of the condition. In fact, it was not until July 2023 that adenomyosis got its own page on the NHS website. However, there is a motivated community of doctors and researchers on a mission to raise awareness of adenomyosis.

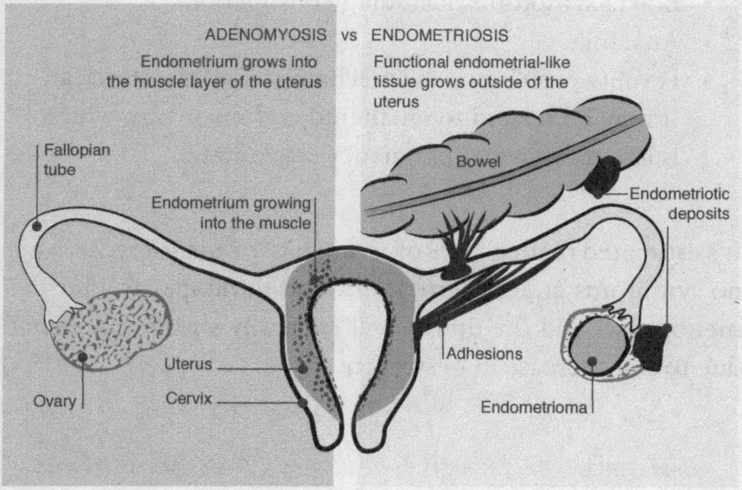

Figure 4.1. *The differences between adenomyosis and endometriosis.*

Symptoms

- Heavy periods.
- Painful periods.
- Bleeding in between periods.
- Painful sex.
- Pelvic pain – often described as a heavy or dragging sensation.
- Pressure symptoms (from the fibroids pressing on other organs).
- Bladder symptoms, including increased frequency, incomplete emptying or urine retention.

- Bowel symptoms, including constipation.
- Anaemia.
- Fertility problems – the mechanism for this is unclear. It may be related to an altered endometrium, which is less receptive to pregnancy implantation.

It's estimated that 20–30% of women with adenomyosis have no symptoms at all.[45] Symptoms tend to disappear after the menopause, and the uterus will generally shrink somewhat due to the decrease in oestrogen.

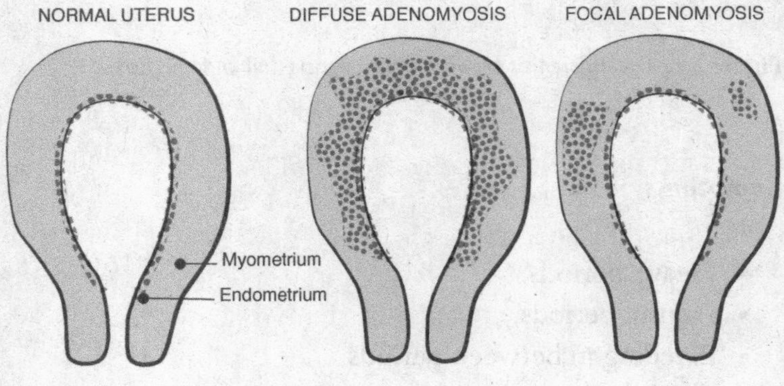

Figure 4.2. *The differences between diffuse and focal adenomyosis.*

Diagnosis

Adenomyosis can be diagnosed on an ultrasound or MRI scan. In some women it may be scattered throughout the entire myometrium (known as diffuse adenomyosis) or seen in discrete areas (known as adenomyomas or focal adenomyosis) (Figure 4.2). Adenomyomas in particular may be mistaken for fibroids at times. Scanning technology, particularly ultrasound, has improved exponentially over the last few decades, which makes adenomyosis easier to diagnose.

I often see patients who have been diagnosed with adenomyosis who have had symptoms for years and have not had any abnormalities found on previous scans. In this situation, it might be either that the woman didn't previously have adenomyosis but does now, or they have always had it but this is the first time it's actually been seen. Prior to the widespread use of scanning technologies, the only way to diagnose adenomyosis was when examining the uterus under a microscope after a hysterectomy. This is one of the reasons we don't know how many women actually have adenomyosis. A study of women attending a gynaecology outpatient clinic found that 20% had ultrasound evidence of adenomyosis, with the highest rates seen in women aged 40–49.[46] Conservative estimates put the figure in the general population to be about 10%.

Treatment options for adenomyosis

There are relatively few clinical trials and studies reporting on the best treatments for adenomyosis. Treatment is aimed at reducing symptoms; unfortunately, a hysterectomy is the only way to get rid of adenomyosis entirely.

Non-hormonal treatments

Painkillers, including NSAIDs and paracetamol – These may be helpful for mild to moderate period-related pain associated with adenomyosis.

Mefenamic acid – This can reduce pain and bleeding, but has no impact on the adenomyosis itself.

Tranexamic acid – This can help to reduce bleeding (which can be a source of pain due to the increased cramping of the uterus to try to eject the blood) but it will have no impact on the adenomyosis itself.

Hormonal treatments

Hormonal coil (Mirena®) – This helps to reduce bleeding, pain and the size of the uterus. This is the most effective treatment, more effective than the COCP.[47] NICE guidelines state that this should be the first-line treatment for heavy periods where adenomyosis has been diagnosed. The coil can also help to reduce any anaemia that results from adenomyosis-related heavy periods.

The combined oral contraceptive pill (COCP) – This can also significantly reduce the amount and duration of bleeding and pain during menstruation. It also reduces the size of the uterus, which is important because an enlarged uterus can be a cause of pain.[45]

Progestogen-only pill (POP), contraceptive implant, contraceptive injection – These may all reduce the amount of bleeding and pain in adenomyosis, but they do not reduce the size of the uterus.

GnRH analogues – These can be very effective in reducing period pain associated with adenomyosis and bleeding; however, the menopausal side effects and the eventual need for 'add-back' hormone replacement are unappealing to most women, so these are usually used as a short-term measure for a few months immediately prior to surgery rather than as a long-term therapy.

Non-surgical procedures

Uterine artery embolisation (UAE) reduces the size of the uterus and reduces bleeding in over 75% of women, reduces pain in 64%, and reduces pressure-related symptoms in 55%.[48] However, there is no good data to say that it's safe to get pregnant after UAE, so this treatment is not recommended for women who wish to get pregnant. (NB: Endometrial ablation can be an effective treatment for heavy bleeding, but this is generally avoided in women with adenomyosis because, while it reduces bleeding, it may make the pain worse.)

Surgery

Hysterectomy – The only way to remove adenomyosis entirely is to perform a hysterectomy to remove the uterus. You may decide to have your ovaries removed at the same time: this will depend on several factors, including whether you also have endometriosis. If you have severe endometriosis, an endometriosis specialist may have to perform your hysterectomy. **GnRH analogues** may be used for a few months prior to surgery to shrink the uterus, which should result in lower blood loss during surgery, and can also reduce anaemia to optimise your health before the surgery.

Excision of adenomyoma – This is not a common procedure. It involves the removal of a specific lump of adenomyosis called focal adenomyosis or adenomyoma, and the procedure may reduce pain and bleeding. This may be performed if medical management has been unsatisfactory and fertility is a priority, making a hysterectomy an unsuitable alternative. Surgery for diffuse disease (disease that is scattered throughout the uterus) is not possible because this would be too damaging to the muscle layer of the uterus, so this is not suitable for most cases of adenomyosis.

Fibroids

Fibroids are benign (non-cancerous), spherical overgrowths of the smooth muscle layer of the uterus. They grow under the influence of oestrogen and progesterone. The medical term for fibroids is leiomyoma, and they can range from pea-sized to the size of a watermelon. Doctors often refer to their size in comparison to the size of a pregnant uterus, so your doctor might write something like 'the uterus is 20 weeks size'. This means your doctor has estimated that your uterus is about the same size as the uterus of a woman who is 20 weeks pregnant.

You can have one, or several, fibroids, and they can grow on their own or in clusters. Fibroids are incredibly common, with at least 70% of women having one at some point, although the true number may be higher because many women have no symptoms so their fibroids are never found. If you don't have any symptoms (which is estimated to be the case in at least 50% of women with fibroids[49]), you don't need to do anything. Black women are up to three times more likely to have fibroids than white women, and in Black women fibroids tend to grow larger and cause problems from an earlier age.[50] The symptoms you may have depend on the size and location of your fibroids (Figure 4.3).

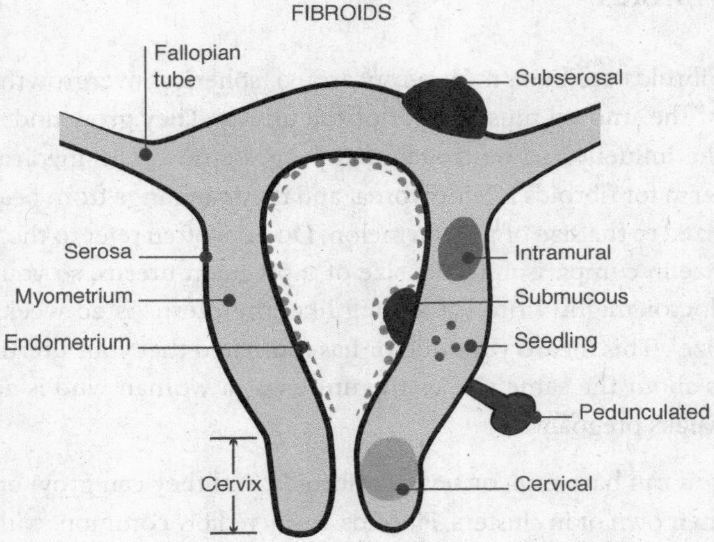

Figure 4.3. *Types of fibroid.*

There are many types of fibroid, and these are discussed below.

Subserosal fibroids are on the outside surface of the uterus. They can sometimes be felt when examining your abdomen as a distinct lump, or several lumps if you have many of them.

Intramural fibroids grow predominantly within the wall of the uterus. These are the most common type, but many women have these without any symptoms.

Submucous fibroids grow directly below the endometrium. These are the type most likely to cause bleeding.

Some fibroids are **pedunculated** – this simply means that they grow on a stalk. You can have pedunculated subserosal fibroids and pedunculated submucous fibroids. They are usually fairly easy to remove, thanks to their stalk.

Seedling fibroids are tiny – often too small to see on a scan. This type of fibroid grows alongside other fibroids. They can grow if larger fibroids are removed, as this gives them access to the supply of blood and nutrients that the bigger fibroids used.

Symptoms

- Heavy periods.
- Painful periods.
- Pressure symptoms:
  - Bladder symptoms, including a sudden urgency to pass urine, needing to go more often, being unable to fully empty your bladder or dribbling urine after going to the toilet.
  - Bowel symptoms, including constipation and haemorrhoids.
- Pelvic pain.
- Pain during sex.

- Anaemia.
- Fertility problems:
  - o Difficulty getting pregnant.
  - o Miscarriage.
  - o Premature delivery.

Heavy periods are the most common symptom related to fibroids, since fibroids increase the surface area inside the uterus and can prevent the muscle contractions that help to stop bleeding. Passing clots and flooding (a sudden gush of blood) are both frequently reported by women with fibroids. Periods often last a lot longer than the average 2 to 7 days and women can become anaemic due to the heavy bleeding (see page 70).

Pain is also a common symptom. It may manifest as painful periods or as generalised pelvic pain because of the pressure from the fibroids. The larger the fibroids, the more likely you are to have other pressure symptoms, which include constipation (from pressure on your bowel) or bladder problems (if they push on your bladder). Pressure symptoms are present throughout the entire menstrual cycle, not just during your period. For some women the pressure of fibroids can even cause prolapse symptoms (see page 58).

It's not uncommon to see women coming to clinic who simply thought they were putting on weight, only to find they have huge fibroids. I once met a yoga instructor with a fibroid that was so large she looked 9 months pregnant – she even had stretch marks. She described finding it increasingly difficult to lie on her front during yoga practice, and assumed that it was down to Covid lockdown weight gain. She must have felt such relief once the fibroid was removed. In spite of its size, it wasn't cancerous, which is understandably what many women are worried about. Having been pregnant with twins, I have a tiny insight into how difficult it must be to have fibroids that press on your bladder and prevent you from being able to eat more than a few mouthfuls at a time. I can't imagine how difficult it must be to go through this for months or even years, like many of my patients have, because my experience was very short-lived, although it didn't seem it at the time!

Diagnosis

Fibroids can be diagnosed on an ultrasound scan. If they are particularly large and/or there are many, an MRI scan may be needed to assess their size and location, and map out their blood supply. An MRI can also be helpful if a doctor is concerned that a fibroid may be cancerous (this is called a sarcoma). This is very rare, with only about 600 cases per year in the UK,[51] but a doctor should suspect this if a fibroid suddenly grows very rapidly, or begins to grow after the menopause, when fibroids should really be shrinking due to lower levels of oestrogen. The risk increases with age from

1 case of sarcoma per 1,250 women who have a myomectomy or hysterectomy under the age of 50, to 1 case per 278 women undergoing the same surgery over the age of 60.[52] The only way to confirm whether a fibroid is cancerous is to remove it and for a pathologist to examine it underneath a microscope.

Treatment options for fibroids

Non-hormonal treatments

- **Tranexamic acid** – To reduce bleeding. This drug has no effect on fibroid size.
- **Mefenamic acid** – To reduce bleeding and pain during your period. This drug also has no effect on fibroid size.

Hormonal treatments

- **Contraceptive pill (COCP and POP)** – While these can reduce the amount of bleeding related to fibroids, thanks to their ability to keep the overlying endometrium thin, they do not help to shrink the fibroids.
- **Hormonal coil** – This can be used if your uterus is not too enlarged by the fibroids, and if you don't have a large fibroid distorting the inside of the uterus, but there may

be a higher chance of the coil falling out (11% fall out in women with fibroids, compared to 3–5% in women without[53]). The coil has been shown to reduce the amount and duration of bleeding because it keeps the endometrium thin, and it can help boost your haemoglobin levels because it reduces bleeding. It has been proven to be so effective that it may reduce the number of women who need to have a hysterectomy due to fibroids.[54] It's not clear whether the coil helps to shrink fibroids, as some studies have shown slight shrinkage while others have shown no change in size.

- **Oral progestins (e.g. Provera/medroxyprogesterone, norethisterone**) – These keep the endometrium thin and thus help to reduce bleeding, but have no impact on fibroid size.

- **GnRH analogues** – These may be given in the lead-up to surgery, to help shrink fibroids and reduce heavy bleeding. They work by preventing the production of oestrogen and progesterone.

- **Depo medroxyprogesterone acetate (Depo-Provera/ contraceptive injection**) – This can reduce bleeding, shrink fibroids, and prevent them from growing.[55]

- **Contraceptive implant** – This can reduce bleeding but does not reduce fibroid size.

Invasive procedures

- **Uterine artery embolisation** – This reduces symptoms and fibroid size.
- **MRI-guided focused ultrasound (MRgFUS)** – This reduces symptoms and fibroid size.

Surgery

- **Myomectomy** – This involves the removal of fibroids, leaving the uterus in place. It can be performed via a cut in your tummy or through the cervix, depending on the location of the fibroid/s planned for removal. This type of operation is generally intended for women who wish to get pregnant in the future.
- **Hysterectomy** – This is the removal of the uterus, and is the only way to entirely prevent fibroids from coming back. Your ovaries could be left in place.

Non-hormonal and hormonal medications can help with bleeding, but there are no great medical treatments to shrink fibroids in the long term. Surgery may involve removing the fibroids or the uterus (see pages 285–7).

Fibroids, fertility and pregnancy

Fibroids *may* make it harder for some women to get pregnant. This depends on their location. They could be blocking the entrance from the fallopian tubes to the uterus, distorting the uterine cavity, preventing a fertilised egg from implanting, or they could disrupt the blood supply to the endometrium. Having said that, most women with fibroids that don't cause any symptoms get pregnant without any trouble, which is one reason for not removing every fibroid we see on a scan.

Studies relating to the impact of fibroid removal are generally carried out on women who are struggling to conceive and/or having fertility treatment, such as IVF. Submucous fibroids are the type most likely to interfere with fertility, so removing these may improve the chance of a successful pregnancy.[56]

The removal of subserosal and intramural fibroids does not appear to have any impact on the ability to get pregnant, but if you have this type of fibroid and are trying to conceive, your doctor will be able to advise you.

Up to one-third of fibroids grow in pregnancy, due to the extra hormones produced at this time, usually in the first trimester. They may also break down as a result of the woman's changing blood supply, which results in severe pain, typically in the second or third trimester.

This is more common in women with fibroids of over 5cm.[57]

If you have fibroids they will be assessed during your pregnancy scans to determine whether they may impact the birth of your baby. If you have particularly large fibroids you might need extra scans in pregnancy to assess the size of your baby, as having large fibroids makes measuring your bump inaccurate.

If you have a fibroid in your cervix, it could block the way out for the baby, in which case you may be advised to have a Caesarean section. However, most fibroids aren't in the way and therefore a vaginal birth is possible. Women with fibroids have a 3–4 times higher chance of needing a Caesarean section: this may be due to fibroids reducing the efficiency of uterine contractions and preventing the baby from moving into the optimal position to open the cervix during labour.[58] Women with fibroids have a higher risk of heavy bleeding after birth, whether they give birth vaginally or by C-section.

If you do have a Caesarean section, it's not advisable to remove fibroids at the same time because there is a much higher risk of bleeding during their removal due to the increased blood supply to a pregnant uterus, compared to a non-pregnant uterus.

Polycystic ovarian syndrome (PCOS)

PCOS is the most common hormonal condition in women during the reproductive years. It affects up to 13% of women worldwide, but rates vary according to ethnicity and geographical location, with some studies reporting up to 27% of women being affected.[59] While the word 'cyst' features in the name, this condition is not the same as the types of cysts mentioned in the box on ovarian cysts on pages 19–22.

We often think of our female hormones working in isolation, when in fact all the hormones in our body talk to one another and act in synergy. The hormonal changes in PCOS are thought to be driven by insulin resistance, which affects the majority of women diagnosed with PCOS. Insulin is one of the hormones responsible for controlling blood sugar, and when your body becomes resistant to insulin, your pancreas reacts by making more insulin. The result is that, in the ovaries, oestrogen is turned into testosterone, which stops ovulation. Periods will thus become very infrequent or stop completely, which is characteristic of PCOS. Progesterone is only made when you ovulate, so women with PCOS have 'unopposed oestrogen', which means oestrogen acting alone without progesterone. This leads to the endometrium becoming excessively thick, which means that when bleeding does occur it is typically quite heavy and with clots. Testosterone is an androgen (a male hormone). Women need it for bone health, brain health and sex drive, but in much lower levels than men. Due to the excess testosterone production that occurs as a result of hormonal changes in PCOS, women may have excess body hair (hirsutism), acne, oily skin and male pattern baldness.

If you want to get pregnant, you need to be ovulating, so PCOS can cause difficulties getting pregnant. Reassuringly, one large study of women who have given birth showed that over 85% of women with PCOS got pregnant without fertility treatment.[60] Unfortunately, many women who are diagnosed with PCOS report being dismissed and told to 'come back when you want to have a baby'. This is a missed opportunity to provide essential health education about the implications of PCOS, which is associated with many other complications than fertility issues. PCOS is associated with a higher risk of high blood pressure, type 2 diabetes, gestational diabetes (which develops in pregnancy) and sleep apnoea. If you have PCOS and want to get pregnant, you should see your GP to discuss a referral to a fertility clinic after 6 months of trying if you're having irregular periods. If you do need help with getting pregnant it doesn't always involve IVF; if you have PCOS, drugs to stimulate ovulation can be incredibly effective.

If you have PCOS your risk of having endometrial cancer is up to five times higher than the risk for people without PCOS.[61] This is because of long episodes of oestrogen exposure without progesterone, due to irregular ovulation. If you have PCOS then you should be having at least four periods per year to reduce your risk of developing endometrial hyperplasia and cancer (see page 139). If you have fewer than four periods, it's recommended that you use either the contraceptive pill, hormonal coil or cyclical progestogens to reduce this risk. PCOS is not clearly associated with a higher risk of ovarian cancer.

Up to 80% of people with PCOS are overweight or obese. The link between PCOS and body weight is complex, and likely interlinked (rather than one simply occurring as a result of the other). If you have PCOS and are overweight, losing just 5% of your body weight has been shown to reduce insulin resistance and androgen levels, improve menstrual regularity and increase your chance of getting pregnant,[62] so your doctor will often focus on weight loss. While calorie-restricted and ketogenic (a high-fat, low-carbohydrate diet that forces the body into a fat-burning state) diets may be effective for weight loss in the short term and can be effective at improving androgen levels and menstrual regularity in women with PCOS, there is very little evidence that they have any lasting, long-term effects. For this reason, I prefer to shift the focus away from weight. I suggest that women adopt a style of eating that is sustainable, enjoyable, and gives their body the nutrients they need to support healthy hormone production and overall wellbeing for the long term. I also recommend that they take up some form of exercise that will help to build lean muscle and look after their heart health.

Some women with PCOS are not overweight. This is often referred to as 'lean PCOS' and these people also usually have insulin resistance[63]; PCOS is not entirely about weight. The treatment options below are relevant for everyone with PCOS and the lifestyle measures are still important because lean women with PCOS are still at risk of PCOS-associated health complications.

Women with PCOS go through the menopause on average 2 years later than women without it.[64] The hormonal changes associated with PCOS do not disappear after the menopause, so it's important to stay active and healthy to try to reduce the risk of complications of PCOS.

Symptoms

- Irregular or absent periods. For a definition, see pages 66–7. Irregular cycles in PCOS tend to be long. Short cycles are uncommon.
- Hirsutism. This is the most common sign of high androgens, and is present in up to 80% of women with PCOS.
- Acne.
- Acanthosis nigricans. Thickened, darker skin may be present in your armpits, on your neck and in skin folds as a result of insulin resistance.
- Male pattern baldness.
- Difficulties getting pregnant.

PCOS symptoms differ according to ethnicity, and are generally more severe, with greater hormonal disruption, in Black and Asian women. It is not properly understood why this is; more research is required in this area.

While these are not typical symptoms of PCOS, higher rates of anxiety, depression and eating disorders have also been noted in women diagnosed with PCOS.[65]

Diagnosis

The Rotterdam criteria were set out in 2003 for the diagnosis of PCOS. They were recently modified to amend the number of follicles required for a diagnosis of PCOS.

To meet the criteria for a diagnosis of PCOS, you need two out of these three symptoms:

1. Absent or irregular periods.
2. Signs of high androgen levels. This may be based on either:
    a. Blood tests – to check levels of testosterone. If testosterone levels are normal and PCOS is still suspected, it is appropriate to check dehydroepiandrosterone (DHEA) and androstenedione, which are part of the same metabolic pathway as testosterone and may also be elevated, or
    b. Hirsutism – quantified using the modified

Ferriman–Gallway scoring system based on the amount and location of body hair.

3. Polycystic appearance of the ovaries – this is defined as having 20 or more follicles on either or both ovaries, or a three-dimensional ovarian volume of more than $10cm^3$. This has been revised due to improvements in scanning technology, and the fact that the previous criteria of 12 or more follicles led to overdiagnosis of PCOS.

As you can see from the criteria above, neither a blood test nor a scan is essential for a diagnosis. Blood tests can be useful to look for other causes of irregular periods, such as thyroid disorders, to check for anaemia (as a result of heavy periods) or to check for diabetes (having diabetes is more common if you have PCOS). You need to stop hormonal contraception for 3 months before having a blood test, as contraceptives will interfere with levels. Blood tests are not terribly useful for monitoring PCOS once it's been diagnosed.

If you're having heavy or painful periods, or bleeding when you're not on your period, an ultrasound scan can be useful to look for causes other than PCOS. It's very common for women to have a scan and be told 'you've got lots of cysts on your ovaries'. This does not automatically mean that you have PCOS. Remember that eggs develop in tiny cysts called follicles. It's very normal to have these cysts as part of the normal function of the ovary, and the diagnostic criterion is very clear: there must be an excessive number present. These cysts are not a *cause* of the disease, but a consequence, so removing them is not going to treat PCOS. These little cysts represent eggs that are stuck in the early development phase within the ovary, but are not able to get to the stage of being released because your body is sending the wrong hormonal signals (a trademark of PCOS). The younger you are, the more eggs you have, and therefore you have a higher chance of your ovaries appearing polycystic. For this reason, ultrasound scanning should not be used to diagnose PCOS during the first 8 years of menstruation, because most teenagers' ovaries will look polycystic and using this criterion leads to overdiagnosis.[66]

Treatment options for PCOS

Treatment is tailored to the individual. It depends on what your main symptoms are, how often you have periods, and what your imminent fertility plans are.

Lifestyle modification – This is important for anyone with PCOS, irrespective of their weight. Exercise and healthy eating play a role in hormone health. Both also reduce the risk of future health complications of PCOS, as discussed above.

Diet – There is no food or food group that either causes or cures PCOS, but eating well is important. My preference is for a Mediterranean-style diet, with plenty of vegetables, legumes (these include lentils, peas, broad beans, chickpeas, etc.), fruits, nuts, wholegrain cereals, olive oil as the main source of fat, moderate amounts of dairy, including yoghurt and cheese, with fish and lean meat and a relatively small amount of red meat or processed foods. This has been shown to be better than low-carb diets for improving insulin sensitivity – and is easier to stick to.[67] A referral to a dietician can be very helpful if you need advice in this area.

Exercise – This helps to make the body more responsive to insulin, and also helps to produce a protein called sex hormone binding globulin (SHBG), which reduces the amount of active testosterone in the bloodstream. This can help to improve acne and reduce excess hair growth, and can result in more regular menstrual cycles.[68] A comparison of high-intensity interval training (HIIT) and weight training showed that they were equally effective for symptom control and improving body composition.[69] The NHS recommendation is a minimum of 2.5 hours of moderate-intensity physical activity per week, or 75 minutes of vigorous exercise, or a combination of the two, including muscle strengthening activities on two non-consecutive days per week.[70] As a guide, during a moderate activity (e.g. brisk walking, racket sports or leisurely cycling) you could hold a conversation, whereas during vigorous exercise (e.g. running, circuit training or spinning) you would find it difficult to keep chatting.

Non-hormonal medication

Tranexamic acid – This can help reduce the heavy periods that are associated with PCOS.

Spironolactone – This is a diuretic that is primarily used for blood pressure control. It has anti-androgen properties which can help reduce the acne and excess hair growth associated with PCOS. This is an 'off-licence' use of spironolactone (see box on page 230), so it would need to be prescribed by a gynaecologist or dermatologist rather than your GP. Other treatments for acne, such as antibiotics and retinoid creams, are usually prescribed by your GP or dermatologist rather than a gynaecologist.

Metformin – This is an anti-diabetes medication that can increase insulin sensitivity and reduce insulin production. It used to be a classic PCOS treatment, but more recent data suggests that it's not as effective as originally thought. It's generally reserved for use in PCOS if you have type 2 diabetes or pre-diabetes: it may improve menstrual regularity and high androgen levels, but it can cause some unpleasant gastrointestinal side effects, such as bloating and loose stools.

Inositols – These are nutritional supplements that work on the insulin signalling pathway. They can reduce insulin resistance, improving menstrual regularity and reducing androgen levels.[71] Inositols are the most promising treatment to emerge in the PCOS arena in the past few years, but there is still some work to be done to find out which type is most effective (myoinositol or D-chiro-inositol). Many doctors are keen to discuss using them because they don't appear to have any serious side effects.

Vitamin D – Up to 85% of women with PCOS have low vitamin D (which may worsen insulin resistance) and high testosterone levels. These can be improved by taking supplements.[72]

Hormonal medication

This is the most common type of medication used to treat the symptoms of PCOS. At work, I have been sad to hear many women say they felt forced to take the pill. This isn't the only option for dealing with symptoms, but there are some crucial safety reasons why doctors recommend it to women with PCOS, and I will explain these here.

COCP – First and foremost, there are safety advantages to taking the COCP when you have PCOS. This is because it provides progestogens to stabilise the endometrium, to reduce your risk of endometrial hyperplasia and cancer,[73] discussed further on page 139. I want to be very clear: taking the COCP doesn't 'reset' your hormones, as I hear some women have been told, because when you stop taking the COCP you will still have PCOS and will likely have irregular periods and the symptoms of high androgens.

However, the COCP can help to improve some of the symptoms of PCOS. They help you to control when you have a bleed rather than waiting for months for a period to come, and when it does the pill will likely make it less heavy and painful. The combination of oestrogen and progesterone is particularly helpful for reducing androgen production by the ovaries, and increases SHBG levels. If you are particularly troubled by these symptoms your doctor may suggest a COCP containing cyproterone acetate, dienogest or drospirenone (which is a derivative of spironolactone) as the progesterone component, due to their strong anti-androgenic abilities, although they are associated with a slightly higher risk of blood clots (see pages 243–5).

Hormonal coil or POP – These are two other options for endometrial protection, but they're unlikely to improve acne and hirsutism in the same way as the COCP, so they could be used with anti-androgen medications such as spironolactone.

Oral progestogens, e.g. Provera (medroxyprogesterone acetate) and norethisterone – These can be taken every few months for 10–14 days. When you stop taking them you will have a bleed, the purpose of which is to reduce the risk of endometrial hyperplasia and cancer. This does not act as a contraceptive.

Polyps

A polyp is a small, fleshy overgrowth of tissue, often on a stalk, on a mucous membrane, which is a moist lining present in many areas of the body including the mouth and bowel as well as inside the uterus (endometrial polyps) and cervix (cervical polyps).

Endometrial polyps are common, more so after the menopause, and are rarely found in women of under 20. There is a small chance of them containing precancerous or cancerous cells: 5.4% after the menopause and 1.7% before.[74] The chance that a polyp may be cancerous is higher if you experience bleeding or have diabetes or high blood pressure.[72] Polyps grow under the influence of oestrogen; if you are taking tamoxifen (a drug used to treat breast cancer) and HRT, you have a higher chance of developing polyps. Endometrial polyps may occasionally be found during investigations for fertility problems. Many women with polyps will go on to have a successful pregnancy. However, some doctors believe they can reduce the chance of a fertilised egg implanting successfully, so if you are due to undergo fertility treatment your doctor may recommend that polyps are removed first.

Cervical polyps are also common, and 25% of women with a cervical polyp may also have an endometrial polyp.[75] The chance of a cervical polyp being cancerous is around 1%, although a large study of women with polyps found that none contained any cancerous cells.[76] Most doctors agree that they don't need to be removed if you're not having any symptoms. They don't appear to interfere with fertility or cause problems for vaginal birth. Occasionally they may cause bleeding during pregnancy, which can lead to anxiety, but removal is not usually recommended during pregnancy (due to the risk of heavy bleeding). They may be removed after your pregnancy if you're still experiencing bleeding.

Symptoms

- Bleeding in between periods.
- Bleeding after sex.
- Bleeding after the menopause.
- Excessive vaginal discharge (cervical polyps only).
- Heavy periods (endometrial polyps only).

It's common to have a cervical or endometrial polyp and not have any symptoms. Cervical polyps are commonly found during a smear test. Endometrial polyps may be found during a scan to look for other problems not related to bleeding (which is the case in 36% of postmenopausal women with polyps and 44% of those who haven't gone through the menopause[77]). If you don't have symptoms, the chance of a polyp containing abnormal or cancerous cells is lower.

Diagnosis

Endometrial polyps can be diagnosed on an ultrasound scan. They may also be found during a hysterosalpingogram (HSG) or a hysterosalpingo-contrast sonogram (HyCoSy) (see page 277) as part of fertility treatment. Some are obvious; some are less obvious, and instead the endometrium appears thickened overall. Sometimes they are mistaken for fibroids.

Cervical polyps don't require any further investigation for diagnosis as they can be clearly identified on speculum examination.

Treatment options for polyps

There is no medication that will get rid of polyps. A minor surgical procedure is required to remove them. They will then be sent to the histology lab to be examined to determine whether they contain any precancerous or cancerous cells.

Endometrial polyps – These can be removed during a hysteroscopy, either in the outpatient clinic if they are small or in theatre under general anaesthetic. A hysteroscopy allows a surgeon to see the entire endometrial lining and examine it for polyps. Occasionally during a hysteroscopy the surgeon finds that the polyp has disappeared on its own – this usually happens after a heavy bleed. Studies show that 75–100% of women who have polyps removed report an improvement in bleeding,[78] although polyps can recur. Using the hormonal coil after polyps have been removed can reduce the chance of recurrence.[79] Further information about polyps containing abnormal precancerous or cancerous cells can be found on pages 139–48.

Cervical polyps – These can easily be removed in clinic if the polyp has a good stalk. If it doesn't, we describe the polyp as 'broad-based'. It might require removal under anaesthetic in theatre.

Endometrial hyperplasia and cancer

Endometrial cancer is a cancer of the lining of the uterus. It is the most common type of uterine cancer (which is also referred to as womb cancer). Cancer can also develop in the muscle layer of the uterus (called a sarcoma), although this is much less common.

In the UK about 3% of women will develop endometrial cancer at some point: over 85% of cases occur after the menopause.[80] Over the past two decades there has been a steady rise in cases of endometrial cancer, especially before the menopause, and obesity is the biggest contributing factor to this. I think it's important to be honest here: the scientific literature demonstrates a clear link. This is because of the ability of fat tissue to produce oestrogen, which drives the development of endometrial cancer. The increase in insulin resistance and higher levels of inflammation also play a role. This is why PCOS, even in women who are not obese, increases the risk of endometrial cancer.

Exercise has been proven to reduce the risk of endometrial cancer for all women,[81] so it's important for us all to incorporate some form of physical activity into our lifestyle, whatever our weight, BMI or body shape. Breastfeeding and taking the contraceptive pill or hormonal coil have also been shown to reduce your lifetime risk of developing endometrial cancer. About 5% of cases are related to inherited genetic mutations, the most common being Lynch syndrome.[82]

While most of us have heard of endometrial cancer, I imagine far fewer people have heard of endometrial hyperplasia. This is an excessive thickening of the endometrium. When it is examined under a microscope, you can see overgrowth of the glands. This happens when a woman has prolonged exposure to unopposed oestrogen without progesterone (e.g. in untreated PCOS, or during the perimenopause and post-menopause). Hyperplasia can be categorised into two groups based on how abnormal the tissue looks under the microscope: hyperplasia without atypia and atypical hyperplasia.

Endometrial hyperplasia is estimated to be three times more common than endometrial cancer. If left untreated, it's estimated that less than 5% of cases of hyperplasia without atypia will turn into cancer within 20 years. With atypical hyperplasia, 8% of cases will turn into endometrial cancer within 4 years, 12% by 9 years and 28% by 19 years.[83] However, about 40% of cases of atypical hyperplasia occur alongside cancer, and that is why hysterectomy is usually the recommended form of treatment. Not all cases of hyperplasia will turn into endometrial cancer, and not all cases of endometrial cancer are preceded by endometrial hyperplasia.

Lynch syndrome

This is an inherited genetic condition that occurs due to mutations in one of the genes involved in repairing damaged DNA. It affects about 1 in 450 people and increases your lifetime risk of several cancers, most commonly colorectal (bowel) and endometrial cancer.

	General population	With Lynch syndrome
Colorectal cancer	6%	80%
Endometrial cancer	3%	50%

There is also a higher risk of cancers of the ovary, pancreas, stomach, bladder and prostate, although to a lesser degree.

In my department at work, we run special clinics for

women with inherited conditions known to increase their risk of gynaecological cancers. Most of the women who are referred with Lynch syndrome have found out about this because someone in their family has recently been diagnosed with colorectal (bowel) cancer. Every patient diagnosed with colorectal or endometrial cancer in the UK is tested for Lynch syndrome, and if this is found your family members can be referred for genetic counselling and can choose to be tested too. This requires a blood test. If you have a parent with Lynch syndrome, your chance of inheriting it is 50%.

Taking aspirin has been shown to reduce the risk of colorectal cancer if you have Lynch syndrome, but it's not clear whether it also reduces the risk of endometrial cancer or the other Lynch-related cancers. Colonoscopy (an inspection of the bowel using a flexible telescope) is offered to people with Lynch syndrome every 2 years to screen for bowel cancer. With respect to endometrial and ovarian cancers, there is not yet any effective way of screening, but research is under way. Many women choose to have a 'risk-reducing' hysterectomy and bilateral salpingo-oophorectomy (removal of the uterus, fallopian tubes and ovaries) once their family is complete. If you have no history of cancer, you can usually take HRT afterwards. Your gynaecologist will discuss this with you.

Symptoms

Endometrial hyperplasia and cancer have the same symptoms, which are:

- **Bleeding after the menopause** – This is the most common symptom of endometrial cancer, reported by 90% of postmenopausal women. Of women with post-menopausal bleeding, about 10% will have endometrial cancer. It doesn't matter how heavy or light bleeding is, or how long it lasts, if you have gone through the menopause but you are having bleeding, make an appointment to see your GP, please and thank you. Other causes of post-menopausal bleeding are discussed on pages 50–1.
- **Bleeding in between periods** – In this case, the chance of endometrial cancer or hyperplasia is 1.3%.[26]
- **Bleeding after sex**.
- **Heavy periods** – The chance of having endometrial cancer in this situation is very low indeed – 0.1%[26] – but this still deserves a mention.

Diagnosis

An examination of your vulva, vagina and cervix is important to look for any abnormalities that may be contributing to the bleeding. A transvaginal ultrasound scan (see page 223) is the next step. It may show a thickened endometrium, polyps, or a mass inside the uterus. Early-stage endometrial cancers or endometrial hyperplasia are occasionally diagnosed by chance when having a scan for a reason other than bleeding. Cervical screening (which used to be known as smear testing) doesn't check for problems with the endometrium, but some cases of endometrial cancer may be picked up after a routine smear if any abnormal glandular cells are found which turn out to be shedding from an endometrial cancer. There isn't currently any screening programme for endometrial cancer in the UK, which is why it's so important to be aware of the symptoms.

If you have gone through the menopause and have any of the above symptoms and have a thin endometrium (confirmed on an ultrasound scan), your chance of having endometrial cancer is very low; another cause is much more likely. If you are still having periods, an ultrasound scan is less helpful because your endometrium varies in thickness throughout your menstrual cycle; instead, you should have a biopsy. This is also the case if abnormalities are found during your scan: you will need to have a biopsy of the endometrium to confirm or rule out cancer or hyperplasia. If the entire endometrium is thickened, a biopsy can be taken in clinic. This is most commonly performed using a Pipelle aspirator. This is like a thin straw that is passed through the cervix, creating its own mild suction to sample some of the endometrium. If there is any evidence to suggest a mass (which might suggest a polyp or tumour) a hysteroscopy should be performed to take a more targeted sample (this is described on pages 272–3). Samples usually take about 2 weeks to be examined in the lab to make a diagnosis.

If cancer is confirmed on a biopsy, you will need to have further scans to determine your treatment plan. An MRI scan is most appropriate to assess how much of the uterus is involved, and whether the cancer has broken through the wall of the uterus. A computerised tomography (CT) scan can be used to look for cancer that has spread to other areas.

Treatment options for endometrial hyperplasia

Treatment depends on the type of endometrial hyperplasia and its risk of cancer.

Endometrial hyperplasia without atypia

The advice here is to watch and wait. In about 70% of cases the hyperplasia resolves on its own without treatment. Further biopsies will be required to confirm whether it has resolved, is still there, or has progressed. You need at least two normal biopsies taken 6 months apart before you can safely be discharged.

Progestogen treatment – This increases the chance of the hyperplasia going away (or regressing) when compared to no treatment. The hormonal coil (specifically Mirena®) or progestogen tablets (e.g. medroxyprogesterone acetate) are usually recommended. The coil is more effective than progestogen tablets at inducing regression, and may reduce the need for a hysterectomy in the future.[84] Treatment should last for at least 6 months. As above, further biopsies will be needed to monitor the effects of treatment, with two normal biopsies required to confirm regression.

Hysterectomy – This is an option if you don't want to, or cannot, take medication, you don't want to undergo further biopsies, the hyperplasia doesn't go away or gets worse and turns into cancer, or you have other medical issues that could be resolved with a hysterectomy.

Atypical hyperplasia

Hysterectomy – Removal of the uterus is the first-line treatment because in this case the cells are abnormal, there is a higher chance of progression to cancer, and there is a 40% chance of cancer already being present. The cervix must be removed to ensure that all abnormal cells are removed.

Fertility-sparing treatment – This may be possible after careful consideration and discussion of the potential risks. Treatment would be carried out in a specialist centre in conjunction with a specialist fertility team. A hormonal coil is used in an attempt to induce regression, after which about 25% of women go on to have a successful pregnancy.[85] Fertility treatment may be preferred over waiting for spontaneous conception, to reduce the length of time that a woman is not using hormonal treatment, to reduce the risk of relapse. Once your family is complete, it is recommended that you have a hysterectomy due to the risk of relapse and future cancer.

Note that endometrial ablation is not recommended in either situation, because you cannot be sure that the abnormality has been completely destroyed and ablation can cause scarring inside the uterus that would make it difficult to take biopsies in the future.

Treatment options for endometrial cancer

Hysterectomy with bilateral salpingo-oophorectomy – This is the main type of treatment offered for early-stage endometrial cancer that is confined to the uterus. It involves removal of the uterus, fallopian tubes and ovaries, and it can usually be performed via keyhole surgery. In some women aged under 45 it may be appropriate to leave the ovaries to prevent a surgical menopause, but this will be explained by your surgeon. In some cases a biopsy of lymph nodes in the pelvis may be taken at the same time, to check for any cancer cells. You may need to go to a specialist gynaecological cancer centre rather than your local hospital for this surgery. In more advanced stages of disease, when it has spread beyond the uterus, a much more extensive surgery may be offered (open surgery rather than keyhole), with the aim of removing all visible disease.

Radiotherapy – This may be required after surgery, depending on the type of cancer that was found, to reduce the risk of it coming back. It can also be used for patients who are too unfit or unwell to have surgery.

Chemotherapy – This may be considered in cases of very advanced disease prior to surgery, or after surgery, if there is disease left behind that could not be removed and depending on the type of cancer.

Fertility-sparing treatments – This may be possible *if* the cancer is found at a very early stage. Regression takes on average 4–6 months, and up to one-third of women will go on to have a successful pregnancy.[85] However, if regression does not happen within 12 months, your doctor will usually recommend abandoning this treatment and proceeding with a hysterectomy. Progestogens may also be used with women who are unfit for surgery.

Hypothalamic amenorrhoea

Hypothalamic amenorrhoea (HA), also referred to as functional hypothalamic amenorrhoea, is a reversible condition in which a stressor such as extreme dieting, exercise, psychological stress or an acute / chronic medical condition interferes with the regulatory pathways to the hypothalamus, which is the area in the brain that controls ovarian hormone production. As a result, less gonadotrophin-releasing hormone (GnRH) is produced, which results in lower levels of LH and FSH releases. The ovary does not receive the signals it needs for ovarian follicles to mature, or for ovulation and oestrogen production. As a result, periods become very light then disappear entirely.

Data from the 1980s (the most recent we have available!) states that HA is responsible for about 30% of cases of secondary amenorrhoea and that it is common among sportswomen, but in my opinion it is becoming increasingly common in the general population. Many women I see with HA are confused about why this is happening, because they don't exercise to the extreme, for example. However, when you explore how many people live today: a few tough workouts per week, maybe they're training for a 'casual half-marathon', they eat a little salad on the go, then get home to find the only food in the fridge is hummus and a few carrots, they get stressed about a work deadline, go to bed late after midweek drinks with old friends, get up early to commute to work . . . All these things are stressors, and together they can easily create a 'perfect storm' that interferes with hormone production. I don't mean to sound condescending here: when I was doing my PhD, I managed to go for several years without a period. I also know that this is not always easy to reverse, but it's important to do so because while your hormone levels are suppressed you're barely making any oestrogen. Over a long period of time, this can have a negative impact on your bone health and can lead to osteoporosis. It's not uncommon for women to be diagnosed with HA after finding that their periods have not returned after stopping the pill: a phenomenon known as post-pill amenorrhoea. This does not happen because the pill has permanently disrupted their hormones; instead, changes in their lifestyle while they were on the pill have disrupted their hormones, but they didn't know that anything was amiss because they were still having bleeds as a result of the pill.

HA also has implications for fertility: you cannot get pregnant if you're not ovulating. But there's no evidence to suggest that HA has any effect on your long-term fertility if you're able to restart your periods.

Symptoms

The main symptom is no periods. Other symptoms include:

- Low energy levels.
- Low mood and increased anxiety.
- Disrupted sleep.
- Hot flushes.
- Low libido.
- Frequent fainting due to low heart rate and blood pressure.

Diagnosis

Hypothalamic amenorrhoea is diagnosed by excluding other causes first, such as thyroid disorders, high prolactin, premature menopause and PCOS. Blood tests can rule out these conditions. With HA, oestrogen levels will be low and LH and FSH levels will be low or within the normal range.

HA is commonly misdiagnosed as PCOS. The ovaries will often appear polycystic on a scan, which can cause confusion, but doing a blood test to find out hormone levels can be useful for differentiating between the two.

Treatment options for hypothalamic amenorrhoea

Lifestyle modification – To reverse HA, you need to reverse the cause. I've heard a lot of very bad advice in this area. 'You just need to stop exercising' and 'You need to eat as much junk food as possible' don't work. The measures that need to be taken are individual to you, and just as there's no set amount of weight loss, for example, that causes HA, there's no set amount of weight gain that's going to reverse it. Remember I mentioned the cumulative effect of things that can come together to result in HA? The same approach can be applied to trying to reverse it. Chipping away at everything in your life that's causing you stress and focusing on good habits – such as exercising, eating well, sleep and relaxation strategies – will help.

Psychological support – While low mood and anxiety can occur in HA, psychological support can be crucial to help with the lifestyle and behaviour changes discussed above. Cognitive behavioural therapy (CBT) has been demonstrated to be beneficial for recovery.[86]

Hormonal treatments

HRT – Low-dose oestrogen and progestogen-containing HRT should be considered. These may also be beneficial for bone health. However, they can provide false reassurance that all is well because your periods will recommence due to the HRT, distracting you from the lifestyle changes you need to make to truly reverse the condition. The same is true of using the COCP, although this is unlikely to be as beneficial to bone health as HRT so it is usually avoided.

Caesarean scar defects

Having a Caesarean section is a very common way of giving birth to your baby: in 2021, 35% of babies were born by C-section in England.[87] After having a Caesarean birth, you not only have a scar on your abdominal skin, but also on your uterus from the cut that is made to deliver your baby. If the scar on the uterus doesn't heal correctly, a pouch can develop inside the uterus at the site of this scar. This is called a Caesarean scar defect (CSD), also known as a 'niche' or 'isthmocoele' (Figure 4.4).

I imagine that, compared to the other causes of period-related problems that I've discussed so far, this is probably the one that most readers will be hearing about for the first time. Due to the increasing number of C-sections, and improvements in ultrasound technology, CSD is something that doctors are becoming more aware of. While we don't know how likely it is that a woman will develop a CSD, studies show that it seems incredibly common,[88] but thankfully the majority don't cause any problems. There's a lot of research under way into this topic to try and improve our understanding and future treatment of this problem. Having a long labour before an emergency C-section, diabetes in pregnancy, and several C-sections can increase your chance of getting a CSD.[89]

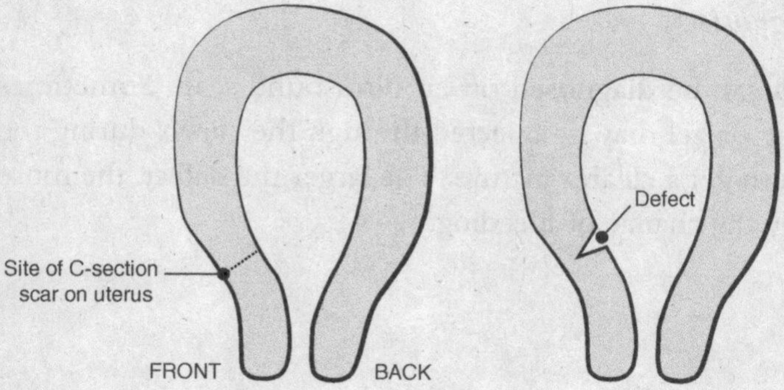

Figure 4.4. *A Caesarean scar defect.*

Symptoms

Many people don't have any symptoms, but if you do, these may include:

- Bleeding – this is thought to be due to menstrual blood becoming trapped in the niche, from where it drains very slowly.
- Periods that stop and start.
- Periods that last a long time.
- Prolonged spotting at the end of your period.
- Brown discharge throughout your cycle.
- Chronic pelvic pain.
- Pain during sex.
- Difficulty getting pregnant.[90]

Diagnosis

CSD can be diagnosed on an ultrasound scan. Sometimes saline or gel may be injected through the cervix during the scan to get a clearer picture. The larger the defect, the more likely the chance of bleeding.[91]

Treatment options

Hormonal

The aim of these treatments is to reduce the overall volume of menstrual blood, and therefore the volume that will get caught in the niche, causing prolonged bleeding.

Contraceptive pill – This may reduce the duration of bleeding and spotting, and can help with pain.[92]

Hormonal coil – This can be very effective at reducing spotting, although it can take up to 9 months to take effect.[93]

Surgery

Repairing the defect via a hysteroscopy, laparoscopy or a combination of the two – This type of surgery is relatively new. In the UK it is only carried out by a small number of experts with a special interest in this field, and is therefore not offered in many hospitals. You may have to be referred to another hospital if this is something that you wish to explore. Small studies have shown that surgery helps to reduce bleeding, although further research is needed to confirm whether it improves the chance of getting pregnant for women who are having difficulty conceiving.[94,95]

Blood clotting disorders

Blood clotting disorders can be associated with heavy periods. These disorders are not related to the formation of blood clots, but rather the opposite: the body is unable to form blood clots, which is necessary to stop bleeding, including during your period. If you have a clotting disorder, you will usually have heavy periods right from your first period.

You may be aware of someone else in your family who has a clotting disorder or a tendency to have heavy bleeding episodes because these disorders can be inherited.

There are a variety of types of clotting disorders. Von Willebrand disease is reported to be the most common bleeding disorder in relation to heavy periods. It occurs as a result of a protein called von Willebrand factor that plays a role in blood clot formation. It is estimated that 1% of the population have von Willebrand disease, but it may be more frequently diagnosed in females due to its relation to heavy periods and bleeding after childbirth. It's estimated to be responsible for 10–20% of cases of heavy periods.[96]

There is also an increased prevalence of bleeding disorders in people with collagen-related disorders such as Ehlers-Danlos syndrome, a condition associated with hypermobility.

While these blood clotting disorders are generally associated with heavy periods, they also come with a higher risk of complications related to ovulation. As previously mentioned, it is common for cysts to develop on the ovaries as part of the ovulation process, and there may occasionally be some bleeding into these cysts which can cause pain, sometimes enough to warrant a trip to A&E, but they usually self-resolve and don't need any treatment. However, some women with blood clotting disorders experience heavy bleeding either into the ovary itself, or into the pelvic cavity from the ovary at the time of ovulation, so if you experience sudden severe pain and feel faint or unwell around this point in your cycle, you should seek urgent medical attention via A&E.

Symptoms

- Heavy periods.
- Heavy bleeding after giving birth.
- Bleeding during dental procedures.
- Frequent bleeding of the gums.
- You bruise easily.
- Frequent nosebleeds.
- Bleeding into joints (if this is happening, you will experience joint swelling and pain).
- Bleeding after minimal or no force/impact.

Diagnosis

Blood tests will be performed to check various aspects of blood clotting.

A haematologist is a doctor who specialises in blood-related conditions. You will be referred to them for further investigations, the formulation of a treatment plan and follow-up.

An ultrasound is also useful to rule out any other conditions that could contribute to bleeding, such as fibroids, polyps or adenomyosis.

Treatment options of blood clotting disorders

Non-hormonal treatments

- **Blood clotting disorder specific treatment** – This will depend on the condition you are diagnosed with and will be determined by your haematologist, in collaboration with your GP or gynaecologist, who will continue to advise on any co-existing gynaecological problems that may be contributing to the bleeding (such as fibroids, polyps or adenomyosis). These problems should also be addressed, and can be treated in the same way as if you did not have a blood clotting disorder. Anaemia that occurs as a result of heavy bleeding must also be treated.

- **Tranexamic acid** – This can be taken during your period to reduce the amount of bleeding.

Hormonal treatments

- **Hormonal coil** – This is recommended as the first-line treatment to reduce the amount and duration of bleeding in women who are not actively trying to get pregnant.
- **COCP or POP** – These are both acceptable alternatives to the hormonal coil to reduce bleeding.

Surgery

This may be necessary if there is a co-existing gynaecological problem. Bleeding during surgery may be heavier than normal as a result of your clotting problem, and your gynaecology team will work with a haematology team to implement measures to reduce surgical bleeding to ensure your operation is performed as safely as possible. In the absence of other gynaecological conditions, endometrial ablation may be appropriate. Endometrial ablation is effective at reducing bleeding in women who have blood clotting disorders and do not wish to get pregnant in the future, although it may not be as successful as it is in women without bleeding disorders. Some women will need to continue medical treatment following the procedure.[97]

Premature menopause

This is referred to in the medical world as premature ovarian insufficiency (POI), or the now slightly outdated term premature ovarian failure (POF). A premature menopause means that a woman aged under 40 has stopped having periods and has very high levels of the hormone FSH: their ovaries have stopped functioning and are no longer releasing eggs on a regular basis in response to the hormonal signal sent out by the brain. Premature menopause is the condition that so many women are understandably terrified of when their periods stop or suddenly become very irregular. Thankfully it's not common, affecting 1% of women under 40, 0.1% under 30, and 0.01% under 20.

Being diagnosed with this condition can be devastating. If you have this diagnosis, there are some helpful resources available, as well as a very supportive online community (see the Resources section, page 315). I also want to reassure you that this is something doctors check for in the routine blood tests we do to assess irregular or absent periods. Surgery to remove the ovaries can also result in a premature menopause (see pages 283–4).

In 90% of cases of POI, no specific cause can be identified. This is called idiopathic POI, although in 30% of cases the woman has a family history of close female relatives, such as mothers or sisters, also having an early or premature menopause. It's worth asking your relatives how old they were when they went through the menopause to get an idea of when it might happen to you. There are no tests that can be done to predict your risk or the age at which you might go through the menopause. Testing FSH or anti-Müllerian hormone (AMH) levels, which is a marker of egg reserve (the number of eggs you have left), or doing an ultrasound scan of your ovaries only gives you a snapshot of what is happening now rather than a forecast of the future. To say 'don't delay having babies' is sensible, but often impractical, advice, because the reasons that people decide to have a baby are complex and multi-faceted. Fertility preservation (by egg freezing) is an option that you might wish to explore. While there is no guarantee that it will result in a baby, it certainly offers an option that wasn't there several years ago, although it may remain inaccessible to many people due to its cost. Egg freezing is currently only available on the NHS to women who are about to undergo cancer treatment (such as chemotherapy or surgery) that will make them infertile or start their menopause.

Where a cause for POI can be identified, these include chromosomal abnormalities (including Turner syndrome and Fragile X syndrome) and autoimmune conditions (including Addison's disease, thyroid disease and type 1 diabetes).

In women with POI the ovaries can occasionally kick back into action intermittently, which can result in ovulation or a random period or even pregnancy. If you have POI there is still a 5% chance of getting pregnant without any kind of medical intervention, so if you don't want to get pregnant you still need to use contraception. Many women are unfortunately diagnosed with POI during fertility investigations, because they've been trying to get pregnant without success. If you have POI you may be able to carry a pregnancy following IVF, but IVF would require the use of donor eggs, because your ovaries will not respond to the drugs used to stimulate them for egg harvesting as they would in someone who does not have POI. In the UK, egg donors must be aged between 18 and 35 and have no serious medical conditions or inherited disorders. Information about egg donors is held by the Human Fertilisation and Embryology Authority, which regulates IVF clinics. This information is currently accessible on request to the individual born as a result of that donation when they reach the age of 18.

Symptoms

- Absent or very infrequent periods for at least 4 months – this is the most common symptom.
- Menopausal symptoms related to low oestrogen, e.g. hot flushes, night sweats, low mood, sleep disturbance, poor concentration, vaginal dryness.

Diagnosis

A blood test should be performed to check FSH levels. These will be very high because the brain is trying hard to stimulate the ovaries but they are not responding so the brain reacts by producing even more FSH. FSH levels are usually over 40iu/l. They should be checked on two occasions at least 4–6 weeks apart.

Further blood tests will be performed to investigate the cause of your lack of periods, and a Dual-Energy X-ray Absorptiometry (DEXA) scan to assess bone density may also be performed, because if you have POI you have an increased chance of osteoporosis.

Treatment options for premature menopause

Since POI is relatively rare in the general population it is managed by menopause specialists, who are either gynaecologists or GPs with specialist menopause training. Treatment is largely based on the use of hormonal medication, with the aim of reducing symptoms and improving long-term health outcomes. The word 'hormone' has a bad reputation: patients often tell me that they 'don't want to take hormones' because of negative things they have read in newspapers and online. Unfortunately, we are rarely taught about the good things that hormones do for our bodies. Oestrogen is so important to our bodies that a lack of it in POI can increase your risk of osteoporosis, dementia and heart disease: replacing the hormones that you lack with synthetic oestrogen aims to decrease your chance of developing these conditions. The British Menopause Society and NICE recommend that hormonal supplementation is used until at least the age of the average natural menopause (51 years). Its use does not increase your risk of breast cancer, when prescribed prior to this age. In fact, women with POI have a lower risk of breast cancer than women without POI.[98]

Hormonal

HRT – This replaces the hormones that are usually made by your ovaries. Combined oestrogen and progesterone is required unless you've had a hysterectomy. There is a lack of research regarding the most effective type of HRT for women with POI, so the decision about which type to use should be based on your preference. HRT does not act as a contraceptive, so you must use additional contraception if you don't want to get pregnant. The POP, implant, or hormonal or copper coil can be used with HRT as well as male or female condoms. The contraceptive injection should be avoided if you have POI because it may decrease bone strength, which may already be low due to POI. There is a safe form of HRT for most women – but if you have had cancer before this may not be the case. A menopause specialist will be able to make recommendations based on your individual situation.

Combined oral contraceptive pill (COCP) – This is effective at managing symptoms for many women, although it may be less effective at protecting bone and heart health over the long term than HRT. Another downside of the COCP is that there is less scope to change doses according to your symptoms, compared to HRT. However, the COCP may be a more attractive option for younger women with POI: they may find it more acceptable to take than HRT because it makes them feel like their peers, many of whom will also be using the COCP. Plus it provides contraception for those who don't wish to get pregnant. Some women may notice an increase in menopausal symptoms during the pill-free week, and if this is the case for you, you can take it continuously (see pages 239–41).

Vaginal oestrogen cream/tablets – These can help with vaginal dryness and discomfort, and can be used with HRT tablets/patches/COCP.

Testosterone – This can be taken to improve libido. Testosterone tends to work better when your oestrogen levels are adequate, so it's common to start oestrogen and progesterone HRT first, altering the dose where necessary, then consider adding testosterone.

Non-hormonal

Vaginal moisturisers and lubricants – These can help with vulval and vaginal itching and dryness, and may be as effective as topical oestrogens.[99] It's important to use one that is designed for vulval and vaginal use and that doesn't contain glycerol, perfumes or parabens, because these may damage the delicate tissue and disturb the healthy bacterial population. Yes Organic is the brand I recommend to my patients. (Note: There is no conflict of interest here; it's just a good-quality brand that has been well scientifically tested).

Vitamin D and calcium – You could choose to change your diet to eat more vitamin D and calcium to help protect your bones. Most people will also need to take a supplement.

Exercise – Weight-bearing exercise (e.g. walking, running, lifting weights, yoga) helps to maintain bone density, and can also have a positive impact on your mental health. There's no one exercise I'd recommend – find one you enjoy!

Psychological support – Receiving a diagnosis of POI can have a significant impact on your mental health. Having POI has been associated with higher rates of anxiety and depression.[100] Talking therapies can be useful to help you come to terms with the diagnosis and to manage your symptoms. CBT in particular has been shown to be effective in reducing hot flushes, night sweats, depression, anxiety, fatigue, and improving overall quality of life.[101]

Premenstrual syndrome (PMS) and premenstrual dysphoric disorder (PMDD)

Around 90% of women experience some type of premenstrual symptoms that alert them to the arrival of their period. These include irritability, breast tenderness, food cravings and mild pelvic cramping (which is a normal response to the hormonal fluctuations of the menstrual cycle). Premenstrual syndrome (PMS) is the name given to these mood-related and physical symptoms, which affect 20–40% of menstruating women.[102] The hallmark of PMS is that these symptoms occur in the luteal phase of the menstrual cycle and disappear in the first few days of your period. The term 'syndrome' means a collection of symptoms that have the same underlying cause: each woman will be affected in their own way. There are over 150 symptoms that make up PMS! While these symptoms are common and relate to the normal hormonal fluctuations in a healthy menstrual cycle, they have long been brushed off as 'just PMS' or 'just part of being a woman', which undermines the significant adverse impact that PMS has on millions of women.

There are also some recognised variants of PMS:

- **Premenstrual exacerbation** (PME) – This means the worsening of an existing medical condition in the lead-up to your period. This may be a psychological condition such as depression or obsessive compulsive disorder

(OCD), or a physical condition such as asthma, epilepsy, migraine or irritable bowel syndrome (IBS).

- **Progestogen-induced premenstrual dysfunction** – This is when a woman has PMS symptoms related to taking progestogen-containing medications.
- **Premenstrual dysfunction with absent menstruation** – This can occur if you're taking medication to stop your periods, but the hormone production that still goes on in your body is sufficient to result in ongoing cyclical symptoms.

Premenstrual dysphoric disorder (PMDD) is a serious form of PMS with more severe emotional and psychological symptoms. It's experienced by 3–8% of women.[103] A startling but very important statistic published in 2021 by the International Association for Premenstrual Disorders stated that 86% of women with PMDD have considered suicide, and 30% report attempting suicide at least once, which demonstrates how seriously we need to take this condition. It must be terrifying to have PMDD – for both the individual and their friends and family. If you are struggling, there is help available from organisations such as Mind or the Samaritans (see the Resources section).

It was only in 2019 that PMDD was added to the International Statistical Classification of Diseases and Related Health Problems (ICD-11), which is a huge step in validating this hugely under-recognised condition. A lack of understanding of PMS and PMDD has led to women being dismissed by doctors and ineffectively treated, if treated at all, and has even led to women being misdiagnosed with bipolar disorder.

Many people don't realise that PMDD is classed as a disability under the Equality Act 2010, which means that your employer should make reasonable adjustments for you at work if you have PMDD. While a lot of the conditions discussed in this book make women dread having their period, PMDD is one of the rare conditions that actually provide sufferers with relief when their period comes. As one patient once told me: 'I feel like I want to kill myself and everyone in sight, and the moment I see blood I think "Halleluiah! It's going to be OK . . . for the next 2 weeks at least".'

As I mentioned at the start of this section, it is normal to have hormonal fluctuations throughout the menstrual cycle, which result in premenstrual symptoms, but these shouldn't have a significant adverse impact on your life and ability to function. There does not appear to be a drastic difference in hormone levels between women with PMS/PMDD and those without, so the most likely explanation is an abnormal sensitivity to hormonal fluctuations.

PMS and PMDD completely disappear after the menopause. However, the perimenopause can be turbulent due to the extreme fluctuations of hormones that take place. While there is very little research being carried out in this area, the consensus among doctors is that PMS and PMDD may worsen in the early perimenopause then begin to dissipate as ovulation becomes less frequent before periods stop for good.[104]

Symptoms of PMS and PMDD

PMS and PMDD have a wide range of symptoms that include, but are not limited to:

Emotional and behavioural

- Depression, feeling low, hopelessness.
- Anxiety.
- Mood swings, increased sensitivity.
- Food cravings.
- Fatigue.
- Reduced concentration, reduced productivity.
- Feeling angry, irritated and annoyed and arguing more with people.

Physical

- Breast swelling and tenderness.
- Bloating.
- Headaches.
- Joint pains.

Diagnosis of PMS and PMDD

Diagnosis is based on the description of your symptoms. The diagnostic criteria for PMDD were first described in 2013 in the *Diagnostic and Statistical Manual of Mental Disorders-5* (DSM-5) of the American Psychiatric Association.[105] These are used internationally. A diagnosis of PMDD requires at least 5 of the 11 symptoms below, one of which must be a core symptom. Keeping a symptom diary is very useful. This must include information about your menstrual cycle, because for PMDD to be diagnosed, there must be a clear correlation with your cycle. You should do this for at least 2 or 3 months – your doctor may give you a questionnaire to complete. The most commonly used is the Daily Record of Severity of Problems, which is a recognised questionnaire to track symptoms of PMS and PMDD. Symptoms must arise in the week before your period, improve when bleeding starts and disappear entirely, or almost entirely, by the week after your period.

Core symptoms of PMDD

- Marked affective lability (this means the tendency to experience strong, variable emotions: e.g. mood swings, feeling suddenly sad or tearful, or increased sensitivity to rejection).

- Marked irritability or anger or increased interpersonal conflicts.
- Marked depressed mood, feelings of hopelessness, or self-deprecating thoughts.
- Marked anxiety, tension, and/or feelings of being keyed up or on edge.[105]

Additional symptoms of PMDD

- Decreased interest in usual activities (e.g. work, school, friends, hobbies).
- Difficulty in concentrating.
- Lack of energy, easily fatigued.
- Marked change in appetite, food cravings.
- Feeling overwhelmed or 'out of control'.
- Changes in sleep (hypersomnia, insomnia).
- Physical discomforts such as breast tenderness, joint/muscle pains, headaches, bloating, weight gain.

No blood tests or scans are required for this diagnosis. However, your doctor may carry out blood tests based on the symptoms that you have reported, to rule out other causes before concluding that you have PMS or PMDD. If there is any uncertainty over the diagnosis, your doctor may suggest using a 3-month trial of GnRH analogue (an injectable medication to induce a temporary menopause). This can be used to test the proposed diagnosis of PMS/PMDD: after the injection, your symptoms should either disappear entirely or significantly improve if you have PMS or PMDD. Once the injections stop, you would go back to having normal periods and would no longer be in a temporary menopausal state.

Treatment options for PMS and PMDD

Lifestyle modification – This is the first thing to try. You may wish to record things like sleep and exercise when you keep a symptom diary, to help you work out if anything specific works well for you or makes you feel worse.

Diet – High-sugar, high-fat diets containing a lot of caffeine and alcohol may worsen PMS symptoms. Eating complex carbohydrates along with plenty of protein may increase serotonin levels and lessen PMS/PMDD symptoms by driving tryptophan, an essential amino acid, into the brain where it is used for serotonin production.[106] Tryptophan-rich foods include whole milk, chicken, tinned tuna, cheese, eggs, bread and oats.

Stress management – Stress may worsen PMS/PMDD, and simply having these symptoms may exacerbate stressful situations, leading to a vicious cycle. It has been shown that women with PMDD may use less productive coping strategies to deal with stressful events,[107] and this is where psychological interventions such as CBT, or even practising mindfulness, may be helpful.

Exercise – Exercise has been shown to increase serotonin levels. Multiple studies have shown that exercise can lead to symptom improvement, with walking, running, swimming and yoga most commonly cited in studies. Exercising three times per week for just 20 minutes each time can also reduce the physical symptoms of PMS, including nausea and bloating.[108]

Non-hormonal treatments

Selective-serotonin reuptake inhibitors (SSRIs), e.g. fluoxetine, citalopram, escitalopram – These are antidepressants that, when used at a low dose, can be very effective, with up to 75% of women with PMDD showing an improvement.[109] This is an off-licence indication. SSRIs can be used during the luteal phase of the menstrual cycle, or continuously. The former may be useful if you are particularly troubled by side effects, such as nausea, loss of libido, sweating and fatigue.

CBT – This can help women learn how to manage their symptoms, and has been shown to be as effective as taking an antidepressant.[110]

Hormonal treatments

The combined oral contraceptive pill (COCP) – There are two types that can be used. They work by preventing ovulation and the fluctuations in hormones responsible for PMS/PMDD symptoms. Taking the COCP continuously without a pill-free week offers further hormonal stability. COCPs containing the progestogen drospirenone have been shown to be particularly effective, particularly for PMDD.[iii] This type of COCP has the highest risk of venous thromboembolism (VTE), although the absolute risk remains incredibly low (see pages 237–8). Other COCPs may also be effective, particularly when taken continuously using one of the tailored methods discussed on pages 240–2.

GnRH analogues with 'add-back' HRT – GnRH analogue injections induce a temporary menopause. If you wish to continue these injections, you should do so using 'add-back' hormones in the form of either conventional oestrogen and progesterone HRT or a medication called tibolone. The purpose of using one of these medications is to reduce the menopausal symptoms associated with the GnRH, and to protect you from bone thinning as a result of the drug-induced menopause.

Surgery

Hysterectomy with bilateral salpingo-oophorectomy – This means removing the uterus, tubes and ovaries. This is not a decision to be taken lightly; it is only considered if all medical therapies have failed. The reason behind this surgery is to remove the ovaries, which will bring on a surgical menopause and stop the hormonal fluctuations of the menstrual cycle, stopping PMS/PMDD permanently. While the uterus doesn't contribute to hormonal fluctuations, it's advisable to remove it at the same time as the ovaries because leaving it behind means you would need to take progesterone as part of your HRT to protect your endometrium. If your uterus has been removed you can use oestrogen-only HRT: this helps to reduce any health complications from years of low oestrogen (which include heart disease, osteoporosis and dementia, particularly if your uterus is removed when you're under the age of 45). Testosterone supplementation may also be required to boost your libido, because the ovaries produce 50% of testosterone in the female body, and lack of this can be profound after a surgical, compared to a natural, menopause. Patients report a high level of satisfaction after having this type of surgery – which shows me what a debilitating disease PMDD can be.

Chapter 5

How can I manage the impact of my periods on my life?

Work and education

An APPG Inquiry in 2017 surveyed over 10,000 women with endometriosis. It found that 23% of respondents had taken time off work because of their period within the last 6 months, and 36% had felt uncomfortable about telling work why they were off.[29] It also showed that 40% of girls and young women reported missing school or university as a result of endometriosis: 55% reported having time off work, 35% experienced financial hardship, 28% had to change or leave their job. This is a problem for individuals, but it's also a problem for the economy that needs to be addressed. Very few companies have a policy on women's health, but I hope that will change over the next few years.

There are some steps that you can take yourself. The first is to have a conversation with your manager, HR or occupational health department, teacher or head of pastoral care. It will probably feel very awkward, but if you never try, you'll never know if things can change. You could ask them whether they have experience of helping other women with similar problems and, if so, what changes they've made to help them, but don't be afraid to make your own suggestions. This could be simple things like having direct access to a toilet, somewhere to keep period products, or the ability to take medications when needed. You could also discuss flexible or remote work or study, and ways to keep in touch if you've been absent. Your manager should also understand that sometimes you will simply need time off. There is often a focus on the impact of absenteeism on the workplace and economy, but in fact presenteeism (loss of productivity while at work) might be an equally weighty burden.[112] You should also discuss what the policy is regarding taking time off for medical care. A hospital appointment can take several hours, and you might have an appointment one day, a scan another day, then a follow-up appointment a few weeks later to discuss the results: this could easily become three whole days off work, depending on the time of your appointment and how far you need to travel. Some hormonal blood tests or scans also need to be done at specific times in your menstrual cycle. These may therefore need to be arranged at relatively short notice. With regards to recovery after surgery, even for a relatively simple process like a laparoscopy you may need a week or two. Now that people are increasingly able to work from home, I have noticed that some of my patients have been pressured to work from home sooner after a procedure than they would if they needed to travel to work. I strongly advise my patients to be firm with their employers and take the recommended time off. If they want to open their laptop earlier than that, great! But give yourself the time you need to recover.

I recommend that you follow up any conversations with your employer or school/college/university with an email thanking them for the opportunity to talk and summarising the problems you are experiencing, the steps you discussed to make your work/education life easier, and any issues that still need resolving. This will ensure that you have something in writing if you run into problems further down the line. With the exception of PMDD, gynaecological conditions are not specifically mentioned under the Equality Act 2010. If you are treated unfairly or lose your job due to problems related to such problems, it may amount to discrimination under the protected characteristics of sex, disability or age (if you are unfortunate enough to have to go down the legal route).

I'm often invited to give talks to organisations to educate staff about gynae health or a specific condition, to help those experiencing it and those working alongside them. If you feel that might be helpful where you work, it's worth reaching out to one of the organisations listed at the end of this book to ask whether they know of any speakers who would be able to do something for your workplace.

Relationships and sex

'A problem shared is a problem halved' is a concept I completely agree with. Talking about gynae health can be tricky, particularly to men, but when you talk about how you feel to your nearest and dearest it can be the first step in making it easier to deal with. Many couples also report that it has strengthened their relationship. If I put myself in the shoes of the person who doesn't have the health issue, I can imagine it must be difficult to know that there's something bothering your partner, but you don't know what it is.

Of course, not all partners are of the opposite sex, and just because someone has never had a period, this doesn't mean that they can't be supportive and understanding. I have noticed some interesting behaviour of men in my gynae clinic. Some sit there looking like they want the floor to swallow them up, in which case I highly commend the woman who persuaded them to join her to support her and hear what we have to say. And on the other end of the spectrum, some men are clearly very involved and will jump into the conversation to provide more information. They often suggest that their partner is downplaying her symptoms; we're all guilty of that! Some men even know the woman's menstrual cycle better than she does, so 10 out of 10 for those chaps!

Talking about period problems to your children is also something I actively encourage, irrespective of their sex. Period education is often referred to as part of 'sex ed' – but remember that gynaecological health is much more than sex. It's part of general health and wellbeing. How exactly you talk to your child and in how much detail will depend on the age of your child and their personality, but I suggest starting simply, by explaining that you're having your period, that you don't feel well and need to rest, or that you're taking tablets because of pain related to your period. You can be guided by your child. If they're interested, I'm sure they will ask you more questions. Of course, you don't want to scare them, but I think demonstrating that it's OK to need some downtime sets a good example of showing respect to our bodies and our health. If you make eye contact with your child and showing that you're open to answering questions, this may help them to understand that they can come to you to talk about worries about their own body. I encourage you to use the proper anatomical terms, such as vagina and vulva, because that's how we can break the taboo of talking about our gynaecological organs. I speak to many women who clearly grew up with mothers who suffered from terrible periods and called their period 'the curse' and other similar names. I don't blame their mothers, of course, because even a generation ago many women did not talk openly about their periods and unfortunately, 'women's problems' have long been dismissed as 'just something women have to put up with', but this can change! We need to open up a conversation about what periods should and should not be like, because that's how we can learn whether what we are experiencing is normal or not.

Painful sex

Period problems and their underlying causes can have an impact on sexual relationships. As you can see from earlier chapters, painful sex is a common symptom of many of the medical conditions relating to periods, and painful sex is estimated to affect 7.5% of sexually active women in the UK,[113] although I think this is a gross underestimate. Addressing this requires open, honest communication. I know this is not easy. I speak to many women who don't feel able to tell their partners that sex is painful for them, so they either avoid sex where possible or just put up with the pain. It may be helpful to describe the pain you're experiencing, whether anything makes it worse or better, and any ideas you have to make sex less painful (such as different positions where penetration isn't so deep, or the woman going on top so she can control the speed and depth of thrusts). It's also important to explain to your partner that sometimes you might need to stop in the middle of having sex. Keeping a note of whether your pain is better or worse at different times in your menstrual cycle and times when sex is more or less painful may be helpful. There are tips on how to talk to your doctor about sex on pages 206–7.

Vaginismus is a common, and likely under-reported, problem that affects sex. It means that the muscles around the vagina tighten involuntarily, making penetration either incredibly painful or impossible. This doesn't just cause problems during sex but also for medical examinations and tampon use – anything that requires vaginal penetration.

The very real physical symptoms that women experience during vaginismus are often influenced by psychological and emotional factors. Previous experiences such as a traumatic examination by a healthcare professional, traumatic childbirth, assault, shame associated with religious or cultural beliefs, gender dysphoria, or being in a controlling relationship can all contribute to pain and discomfort. I see this in a lot of women with conditions such as endometriosis, that cause them a great deal of pain. Often the brain associates penetration with pain, and therefore tenses the pelvic floor muscles as a form of protection. Treatment is very varied, based on the individual, and can include the use of vaginal dilators and wands, pelvic floor physiotherapy, psychological therapies and sexual counselling.

A lot of women report an increase in libido around the time of their period. Period sex seems to be quite divisive – you either love it or hate it. A survey of 2,000 women by Bodyform showed that 51% had engaged in sex during their period.[114] From a health perspective, there is no problem with having sex during your period. I think part of the taboo relates to the fact that period blood is commonly thought of as dirty, which it is not.

Some people believe that having sex or masturbating during your period may help reduce period pain. This may be due to the release of endorphins, which can serve as natural painkillers, and orgasm may temporarily distract the pain-producing nerve fibres. But some women have such painful periods that they don't even want to consider having sex or masturbating, which is completely understandable.

You must remember to use a condom if you are having sex with a male partner, not using any other form of contraception, and you don't want to get pregnant, because it is possible to be fertile during your period, particularly if you have a short or unpredictable cycle. Even if you don't, there's always a chance that you could ovulate earlier than expected. There is also a slightly higher chance of catching an STI from an infected partner during your period because of changes to the immune system of the cervix and vagina. If you're not keen on period sex and you have prolonged bleeding or unpredictable cycles this can result in relationship issues: this is another reason that being able to communicate with your partner is helpful.

Chapter 6

Are there any non-medical interventions I can use?

I am a firm believer in combining conventional medication and treatments with lifestyle modifications; I don't think that you need to pick one or the other. Just as your lifestyle is not the cause of your symptoms, changing it is unlikely to completely cure any gynaecological conditions, but making small changes to your lifestyle could have a hugely positive effect on your health and on how you feel.

I often hear people voicing their frustration that doctors rarely recommend supplements or herbal medications. Lots of people have had a good experience with them, but here I'd like to explain my stance on this. As doctors, we have a responsibility to our patients to ensure we are recommending a treatment that is effective and safe. Pharmaceutical companies must put their drugs through rigorous clinical trials as part of the regulatory process to determine their effect and side effects, then further real-world evidence is required before a drug can be licensed for use. However, the production of supplements and natural remedies is unregulated, so less stringent data about them is available. Studies detailing their effects are often very small, which makes it less likely that the studies are accurate or that they will have a beneficial effect on everyone. I don't want to recommend something that doesn't actually work, that wastes your money, and that may in fact cause harm. As I was once taught, 'if something has an effect, it most likely has a side effect': just because something is natural, this doesn't mean it's harmless.

But of course you may decide to take one of these supplements. If you do, please tell your doctor what over-the-counter medications and supplements you are taking.

Here are some non-medical interventions that I often discuss with my patients.

Nutrition

I'm not a dietician or nutritionist, and I have no specialised training in nutrition. While I've read extensively around the subject, this does not qualify me to give specialist nutrition advice. However, not everyone has access to a professional trained in nutrition, so I try to offer my patients some general evidence-based advice – in a bid to prevent them falling down an online rabbit hole!

The basics

I know it might sound boring, but it really is all about the basics. There are no foods or nutrients that can cause any gynaecological conditions, and unfortunately there aren't any that can cure them either. Fad diets are everywhere, making bold health claims, and while you may lose weight in the short term, any weight loss achieved through extreme measures is unlikely to be maintained. This results in your weight yo-yoing, which has been shown to be detrimental to long-term health. The topic of weight loss is quite sensitive and triggering for many; I prefer to focus on making a long-term commitment to adopting a healthy way of eating that is sustainable, enjoyable, and provides my body with all it needs to keep it working normally. A famous professional sportswoman once said to me, 'If you put crap into your body, you're going to feel like crap.' A pretty snappy summary of what I'm trying to say!

We often hear the term 'well-balanced diet'. To me, the best example of this is based on the Mediterranean diet. I prefer to see this as a style of eating rather than a diet. It's based on eating lots of fruit, vegetables, nuts, seeds, legumes and wholegrains, with olive oil as the main source of fat, moderate amounts of fish, dairy and lean meats and a small amount of red meat. It doesn't require any tracking of calories or weighing out of ingredients, but as a guide your plate should be 50% veggies, 25% protein (such as fish, lean meat, legumes and dairy), with 25% grains, rice or pasta. The more colourful your food, the better, to ensure you get a good mix of all the micronutrients you need.

A few words on some important dietary components and micronutrients

What works for one person may not work for another. One patient might say there's something they absolutely cannot eat because it makes their endometriosis flare up, whereas my next patient says it's their favourite food! If you find that eliminating a specific food or food group from your diet makes a difference to your symptoms, that's great! But if you find no difference whatsoever, please don't feel you need to continue to cut it out: restricting what you eat unnecessarily is hard work and can lead to nutrient deficiencies.

PCOS and endometriosis are the most studied gynaecological conditions when it comes to nutrition.

Dairy – This is often blamed when a woman develops endometriosis or PCOS, but dairy has not been shown to increase the risk of either condition. On the contrary, in fact: in a meta-analysis of studies looking at dairy consumption and endometriosis, women who ate three or more servings per day were less likely to have endometriosis, and cheese consumption had a particularly protective effect.[115] With regard to PCOS, dairy as a whole doesn't seem to have an impact, but low-fat dairy products may increase testosterone levels, prevent ovulation[116] and worsen acne.[117] Remember that dairy foods are a rich source of calcium, vitamin D and iodine, so they are important for overall health. All the evidence suggests that you can enjoy dairy foods without worrying that you're doing something detrimental for your PCOS, but it may be better to choose full-fat versions over low-fat products. If you do plan to cut out dairy entirely, then you should seek nutrition advice to ensure that you're not putting yourself at risk of a deficiency.

Fibre – We should all eat 30g per day of fibre. Most of us don't eat enough, but think we do, because we consume caffeine which helps us to open our bowels, so we don't get constipated. Fibre helps to reduce the chance of constipation, but plays a key role beyond that in maintaining a healthy gut microbiome. This helps to modulate inflammation and oestrogen metabolism, which are two crucial mechanisms for many gynaecological conditions. An altered gut microbiome has been detected in studies of women with endometriosis,[118] fibroids,[119] PCOS[120] and PMS,[121] and in mice with adenomyosis.[122] While this is very early data and doesn't prove any causal link between the bacteria and disease, or prove that modifying our gut microbiome will change our risk of these diseases, or our symptoms, it adds to the list of reasons to add fibre to our diets.

Gluten – Overall there is no evidence that cutting out gluten will improve any gynaecological conditions. If you have coeliac disease (an autoimmune condition in which your body attacks its own tissues when you eat gluten) you have a higher chance of endometriosis. This may be related to the fact that both diseases are related to alterations in the function of the immune system, and chronic inflammation.[123] Symptoms of coeliac disease include abdominal pain, bloating and diarrhoea – the same symptoms that many women experience with endometriosis.

Iron – Iron deficiency is the most common nutrient deficiency worldwide, largely due to heavy periods. It's discussed further on page 70. Once you become iron-deficient it's usually not possible to rectify this through diet alone; you will require an iron supplement. But you should also focus on eating plenty of iron in your diet. Apart from red meat, other great sources of iron include eggs, beans, lentils, leafy green vegetables (e.g. spinach and broccoli), fortified bread and breakfast cereals. One of my favourite ways to make vegetables tastier is to serve them with a squeeze of lemon juice, which contains vitamin C, which helps the body to absorb iron.

Iodine – Iodine is necessary for thyroid hormone production. Deficient or excess thyroid hormones can interact with ovarian hormones and cause problems with menstruation. Low thyroid hormone levels are more common in women than men. While this is largely due to autoimmune reasons, it's important that we all consume enough iodine to support healthy thyroid function. The main dietary sources of iodine are dairy, seafood, seaweed and iodine-enriched salt. Cow's milk isn't naturally rich in iodine, but contains high levels because dairy equipment is disinfected using iodine-based products and dairy cows are often fed an iodine-supplemented feed. Some non-dairy milk alternatives contain added iodine, but if you are vegetarian or vegan there is a reasonable chance that you're iodine-deficient (this is becoming more common in the UK). The British Dietetic Association has a very helpful section on iodine on its website. If you are vegetarian or vegan, or you don't eat dairy or seafood, I suggest you take a look.

Eating around your menstrual cycle

A trend is emerging around eating based on the phase of your menstrual cycle. I'm a great advocate of being aware of your menstrual cycle and learning how you feel at particular times of your cycle, but I fear that letting your cycle dictate your diet could be the newest form of disordered eating. While our hormones do have an influence on how our metabolism works, and our hormones have an impact on our cravings, this is only part of the picture. About half of women aged 16–49 use hormonal contraception, and therefore won't have the same kind of hormonal cycle as women who don't. From a practical point of view, this diet could be tricky to implement in our already hectic lives. However, if you choose to tailor your diet to your menstrual cycle, because you find this helps you, that's great, but don't let it take over your life. Eating should be enjoyable, not a chore.

Intermittent fasting

There are various styles of intermittent fasting, but there is no data to suggest that it helps any gynaecological conditions. Some women find it helps to reduce pain (this may be because the bowel gets a rest), but it may be more beneficial to find a diet that helps more of your symptoms, including bloating, which can contribute to pelvic pain. Keeping a diary of what you eat, and symptoms, and working with a dietician or nutritionist may be beneficial.

Sleep

Lack of sleep doesn't just make you tired and cranky the next day; it can actually have a knock-on effect on your hormones. Your body sees a lack of sleep as a stress factor, which can result in irregular menstrual cycles. Sleep deprivation can also increase insulin resistance, and is especially bad news if you have PCOS, because PCOS is related to insulin resistance. So if you're not sleeping well and you have PCOS, it may worsen the insulin resistance and your symptoms.

Your menstrual cycle itself can affect your sleep. Disrupted sleep is most common during the luteal phase, which may be linked to a subtle temperature rise during this time. Many women also find that they can't sleep during their period – due to pain, needing to get up and change their period products, or night sweats (which can occur because your oestrogen is at its lowest at this time of the cycle). Lack of sleep can worsen PMS and PMDD.[124]

Here are some tips for improving your sleep:

- Aim for a consistent bedtime and wake-up time every day.
- Have a bedtime routine, such as having a shower, a cup of herbal tea and reading a book before bed. This is an opportunity to wind down and tell your body it's time to go to sleep.
- Have a 'caffeine curfew' (the time you stop drinking coffee) of around lunchtime. Caffeine has a half-life of about 6 hours, so if you drink a coffee at 4pm, it's like having half a cup of coffee at 10pm, because half the caffeine is still in your system. Without caffeine, you're likely to find it easier to drop off to sleep and you'll have a better quality of sleep.
- Make a list of things you need to do the following day, or anything that's happened during the day that you're worrying about, to try to prevent your mind racing as you try to fall asleep.
- Avoid screens for at least 90 minutes before bed (the blue light produced by many electronic screens stops the brain from producing melatonin, so we find it harder to fall asleep).
- Avoid big meals shortly before bed.
- Avoid using alcohol to help you sleep – it might help

you to fall asleep quickly, but you will have a poorer quality of sleep and you might even wake up in the middle of the night.

Exercise

Staying active is very important for your overall health and wellbeing, but having period-related problems can certainly have an impact on your motivation to exercise.

The NHS recommendations regarding exercise state that adults should aim to:

- Do strengthening activities that work all the major muscle groups (legs, hips, back, abdomen, chest, shoulders and arms) on at least 2 days a week.
- Do at least 150 minutes of moderate intensity activity per week or 75 minutes of vigorous intensity activity per week.
- Spread exercise evenly over 4 to 5 days a week, or every day.
- Reduce the time they spend sitting or lying down, and break up long periods of not moving with some activity.

Numerous studies have shown that exercising three times per week, for 45–60 minutes at a time, can have a really positive effect on period pain,[125] but remember you need to do this for the whole month. It's safe to exercise during your period. While some people love it and find that it helps with cramps, bloating and general wellbeing, it's absolutely fine if you really don't fancy it. If you're troubled by heavy bleeding, then black leggings are your safest option. Wearing period pants with a tampon or menstrual cup can help you feel more confident if you're worried about leaks.

Remember that exercise doesn't have to take place in a gym – and even things like housework and gentle walking count as exercise. I'm often asked, 'What's the best exercise for X, Y or Z?' and my answer is, 'The one that you enjoy'. There's no overwhelming evidence that any specific form of exercise helps any specific gynaecological condition, but if you enjoy exercising, that will make you stick to it – and that's beneficial for your overall health.

Your menstrual cycle can have an impact on how your body performs during the month. Broadly speaking, during your period you may find high-intensity interval training (HIIT) workouts easier than at other times, because your hormones at this time make your body more able to supply your muscles with the glucose it needs for HIIT training. As oestrogen levels rise, so does muscle strength, making you most likely to get a heavy lifting personal best around ovulation (when oestrogen peaks). After ovulation, your body is most efficient at burning fat, potentially making it the best time to engage in endurance sports such as a long cycle or run. However, this isn't the case for everyone, and there are other factors to take into consideration when it comes to performance, including how well you've slept, eaten and hydrated, and even what kind of mood you're in, so don't feel that you have to structure exercise around your cycle unless you want to. Rather, bear your menstrual cycle in mind if you have a rough session.

Even elite athletes are affected by their menstrual cycle. Jess Warner-Judd posted on social media after the London Diamond League meet on 23 July that she didn't race as well as she wanted to because she had her period. Also, bear in mind that women are more prone to injury at certain times of their cycle.

If you want to be more active – and to stay active – it takes a bit of organisation to begin with. Over time, it will fall into place. Planning when you're going to exercise and what you're going to do can help you work out when you have time.

If you plan to exercise in the evening but always come home exhausted, it's probably not going to work. Could you exercise in the morning? Getting my kit and work bag ready the night before definitely helps me. Remember that walking is also exercise – if you live too far from work to walk there, you could consider parking further away or getting off public transport a few stops early and walking the rest of the way, or going for a walk during your lunch break. If evenings are your time, keep hydrated throughout the day, and have an after-work snack to fuel you. A banana, apple or nuts are my favourite, but I have been known to dive into the ward's chocolate stash . . . sometimes you just need to! Having dinner ready in the fridge for when you get home also helps make your evening more manageable and less tiring. And if you're exercising on your way to work, prepping some breakfast (such as overnight oats or a smoothie) is also a great idea. I often prep my smoothie the night before and just add ice and blend it before I leave in the morning.

Transcutaneous electrical nerve stimulation (TENS) machines

High-frequency TENS machines have been shown to be effective at reducing period pain.[126] These machines are attached to your body using small sticky electrodes over the areas where you experience pain, and a small electrical current stimulates the nerves. You may feel a slight tingling sensation when you're attached to a TENS machine. There aren't any significant side effects, although the sticky electrodes can irritate your skin. At a recent endometriosis event, I met one of the founders of a company called Myoovi, which is a discreet TENS machine developed specifically to target period pain. While I haven't seen any published data on this device, the founder was surrounded by women with endometriosis giving glowing feedback about his product, so I would recommend looking into it, based on their comments.

Chapter 7

When should I seek help?

And what information will my doctor need to help me with my periods?

I always tell people, 'If it bothers you, bother someone about it.'

Health is a very individual issue, and what bothers one person may not bother the next, so it's difficult to set thresholds to determine when you should seek professional help. Instead, I've put together this list to give you a general idea of when you might want to seek help (but the list is not exhaustive):

- Bleeding – passing large clots, leaking through clothing, changing period products every 1–2 hours, having to get up in the night to change period products.
- Any spotting or bleeding between periods.
- Periods that last more than 7 days.

- Periods that are irregular (i.e. you cannot predict when the next one will come).
- Pain – this is very subjective. My general rule is to seek help if you're taking over-the-counter medications such as paracetamol and ibuprofen but these aren't working, or if you're clock-watching to see when you can take the next dose.
- Severe mood changes associated with your menstrual cycle.
- Any symptoms that interfere with your daily life.

Where to seek help

In England you will need to see your GP before you can be seen by an NHS gynaecologist. Your GP will discuss your symptoms with you, perform an examination (where appropriate), and may carry out some investigations, such as blood tests or scans. Where possible, they will start some form of treatment.

GPs are very good at carrying out these initial steps, and in many cases these will be sufficient to treat your problem. Some people are worried about accepting treatment from their GP without seeing a gynaecologist. I want to reassure you that any medications or treatment your GP prescribes will not affect any investigations that we may do in hospital. Since waiting times for a gynaecology outpatient clinic appointment can be very long, I recommend considering your GP's suggested treatment, which should reduce pain and any unpleasant symptoms. Plus, of course, we often suggest the same initial treatment as your GP would.

If your GP's initial management plan doesn't work for you, they're not sure what the problem is, it's complex, or it may need more specialised treatment or surgery, your GP will refer you to a gynaecologist. Occasionally the GP might phone the on-call gynaecology team in their local hospital if they need immediate advice. If they think that you need urgent attention, they will arrange for the on-call gynaecology team to see you in A&E the same day.

You can also go to A&E yourself if your problem is very urgent: this includes very heavy bleeding that's making you feel unwell, or severe pain that isn't relieved with painkillers. When you arrive, you'll see a highly skilled A&E nurse who will decide whether you need to see the doctor immediately or whether you can wait in the queue. Arriving by ambulance does not automatically mean that you'll be seen more quickly. You'll be seen by an A&E doctor who will take a history, arrange any relevant investigations, and start any urgent treatment you need. They may then call the on-call gynaecologist for advice regarding further management. The gynaecologist may come and see you to discuss this, or to discuss admitting you to hospital for treatment. Unfortunately, going to A&E is not the way to get a long-standing problem fixed more quickly: if your problem doesn't require treatment on the same day, you will need to come to see a gynaecologist at their clinic, and for that you'll still need to see your GP for them to refer you.

What is a gynaecologist, and what do they do?

A gynaecologist is a medical doctor trained in diagnosis and treatment of disorders and diseases of the gynaecological organs: the vulva, vagina, cervix, uterus, fallopian tubes and ovaries. They deal with conditions such as period problems, hormonal issues (including PCOS), issues caused by the menopause, prolapses, fertility issues, ovarian cysts, endometriosis and gynaecological cancers. We provide both medical and surgical treatment. In the UK it takes a minimum of 9 years from finishing medical school to becoming a fully qualified gynaecologist. This includes 2 years of foundation training, which is a general postgraduate training scheme undertaken immediately after graduation from medical school. It involves working in several specialties – for me, for example, this included orthopaedic surgery, cardiology, colorectal surgery, obstetrics and gynaecology (O&G), A&E and working in a GP surgery. After these 2 years, doctors apply via a competitive application process to access further training in their specialty of choice. For someone wishing to become a gynaecologist, this is the field of O&G. In the UK, gynaecologists complete a 7-year dual training programme in obstetrics to provide care to pregnant women during their pregnancy, labour and birth, as well as gynaecology. Our training is overseen by the Royal College of Obstetricians and Gynaecologists. Towards the end of this 7-year training programme, there is the opportunity to undertake further training in specific areas of interest related to gynaecology, including keyhole surgery, colposcopy (examination of the cervix if you have an abnormal smear result) and hysteroscopy. Some doctors may spend more time training to develop further specialist skills, such as complex endometriosis surgery and specialist gynaecological ultrasound scanning. There are also four optional 3-year sub-specialist training programmes that doctors can take on top of the core training. These are: gynae oncology (which includes training in complex surgery for gynaecological cancers), urogynaecology (treatment of bladder and pelvic floor problems, including incontinence and prolapse), reproductive medicine (which includes managing fertility problems, including IVF) and fetal and maternal medicine (caring for pregnant women with complex medical conditions, pre-existing or developing during pregnancy, as well as complex pregnancy scanning). After completing O&G specialist training, some doctors will work in both obstetrics and gynaecology, while some will choose to work purely in obstetrics and others in purely gynaecology. As you can see, the training is long. Given the diversity of problems that can be encountered in gynaecology, alongside our core knowledge and skills we all develop our own niche interests along the way. In the UK gynaecologists are not trained to investigate or treat breast problems (as they are in some European countries).

When should my GP refer me to a gynaecologist?

In most cases there is no hard-and-fast rule. The only exception is if a GP suspects a gynaecological cancer. In this situation you would be referred via the suspected cancer pathway for a Two-Week Wait appointment, which means you should be seen by a specialist within 2 weeks of your GP sending the referral. The aim of this is to investigate and diagnose a cancer as early as possible and start treatment promptly. In the majority of cases, of course, we confirm that the diagnosis is not actually cancer, so patients are reassured.

Other reasons to be referred to a gynaecologist include, but are not limited to:

- Symptoms that don't get better with lifestyle changes or medications prescribed by your GP.
- If you'd like to discuss surgery.
- Concerns regarding fertility. (Note: Certain criteria need to be fulfilled before your GP can refer you to a fertility team. One is the length of time you have been trying to conceive, which is usually 12 months up until the age of 35 or 6 months after that.)
- Suspected or confirmed deep endometriosis or endometriosis outside the pelvis.
- Management of premature menopause (menopause before the age of 40).

How to describe your symptoms

My advice is to keep it simple. It's helpful to think beforehand about specific symptoms you want to mention. You should describe how often you're experiencing the symptom, how bad it is, and if there's anything you've tried that makes it better or worse. When explaining the severity of the symptom, it can be helpful to say what it is stopping you from doing in your day-to-day life. It is useful to say if you are worried that it might be a particular condition, but it doesn't matter if you have no idea; it's our job to work that out.

You don't need to use any fancy terminology, but it is helpful to learn the proper words for your anatomy. The Eve Appeal, a gynaecological cancer charity, does a lot of great work to educate the public about the basics, so check out its website. If you feel more comfortable using slang terms, that's also absolutely fine and you won't be judged for it, but the gynaecologist you see will probably check with you that you're both talking about the same place. If you're struggling to describe what or where you feel pain, for example, sometimes it's easier to say, 'Please can I show you what/where I'm talking about?' This can be the most effective way of communicating a problem.

Talking about sex

This topic deserves its own box because I want to emphasise that it really is OK to talk about sex in a consultation with a gynaecologist, but I know it may seem daunting. I feel that both patients and doctors are sometimes reluctant to prioritise sex as a pleasurable experience. In medical consultations, I find that women only bring up problems with sex if they want to get pregnant. Realistically, most of us are having sex for pleasure, rather than baby-making, the majority of the time, so please don't feel guilty for wanting to have sex that you actually enjoy.

When I talk about 'sex', I don't just mean heteronormative penetrative sex, which may not be the type of sex that you're having. It's OK to discuss having sex with same-sex partners, masturbation, using sex toys, or having multiple partners. Your doctor should not judge you based on your sexual orientation or preferences.

While you don't have to talk about your sex life if you don't want to or you don't think it's relevant, in a gynaecological consultation we will usually ask you if you are sexually active and, if so, whether you have any pain or bleeding associated with sex.

Here are some suggestions for things you may wish to tell your doctor about sex, that may be helpful for them to know:

- If you bleed during or after sex . . .
  - How often it happens, e.g. every time, just once
  - About the colour of the blood, e.g. fresh red, brown
  - Approximate amount, e.g. is it just on wiping, or do you need to wear a pad?
- If you have pain during sex . . .
  - How often does it happen? Is there any link to timing in your menstrual cycle?
  - Location of the pain, e.g. on the outside, deep inside
  - Whether it's associated with any vaginal dryness or irritation
  - Whether it's linked to orgasm
- Problems related to libido
- Anything else about your sex life that is bothering you!

Cycle tracking

I thoroughly recommend cycle tracking – by which I mean, keeping track of when you have your period, how heavy or painful it is, and any other symptoms that you have throughout the month (such as bloating, mood swings, headaches . . . the list is endless). I can barely remember what I had for dinner last night, so there's no way I could remember the date and timings of my symptoms over the last month, never mind the last few months.

When I'm seeing a patient in clinic, I'm absolutely delighted when they whip out a diary of their menstrual cycle! It really helps me to understand exactly what is happening, and when. Tracking can involve using an app, the calendar function on your phone, or a good old-fashioned paper diary.

Keeping a diary can be helpful for several reasons. It can help you recognise whether:

- You're having a regular menstrual cycle.
- You're having recurring symptoms – and, if so, how often.
- Your symptoms are related to your menstrual cycle.
- Any lifestyle changes you make or treatment you use is having any impact.

How to advocate for yourself

This is the section I really wish I didn't have to write. However, in 2021 the Department of Health and Social Care launched a call for evidence regarding women's experience of receiving healthcare in England. Out of almost 100,000 responses, 84% of women reported that there had been times when they had not been listened to by a healthcare professional.

This is an astounding statistic. As a doctor, I find it incredibly embarrassing: as a medical profession, we must do better. Here I'd also like to reassure you that there are a lot of very caring healthcare professionals out there who do want to help you, so please persist. Your health and wellbeing are important.

If you feel that you're not being listened to, or are being dismissed, here are some suggestions of questions to ask:

- Ask what is causing your symptoms.
- If you are concerned that you have a specific condition (e.g. endometriosis), explain this. If the doctor does not agree, ask them to explain why.
- Ask whether the doctor thinks further investigations may be helpful and, if not, why not.
- Explain that you are not happy to keep going with these symptoms, and ask what they suggest you do next.

There may be a good reason why your doctor doesn't consider a specific test or referral to be helpful, and if this is explained it will help you to understand their reasoning.

Taking someone with you to the appointment is also useful, because we all hear different parts of a conversation, and if you're worried it can affect your ability to listen and take in information. Also, having a friend or advocate there might make you feel more confident about speaking up. It's really important that you do so during your appointment if you're not happy, because sometimes the cause can be a simple misunderstanding that's easily rectified.

If you are still not receiving the help you need, you can ask to see a different GP – or if your appointment is at a hospital, ask to see a different doctor in the clinic.

If you are still not satisfied, contact the GP practice manager or, in a hospital, the Patient Advice and Liaison Service (PALS).

How to prepare for an appointment with a gynaecologist

It can be overwhelming to think about going to see a gynaecologist about a problem that's been bothering you. Writing down some notes can be helpful: to help you get through a lot of information quickly and effectively, and as a prompt if you get flustered. The gynaecologist will be guiding the conversation, but I've listed here the types of things we will be asking you, so you can think about these beforehand:

- What are your symptoms?
- How do they impact on your quality of life? E.g. can you go to work/school? Can you do the things you enjoy in your spare time? Is your sex life affected?
- What have you tried so far to help relieve your symptoms? (It's worth writing down a list of the medications you take, because electronic note systems between your GP and the hospital and between hospitals are notoriously difficult to link, so we often do not have access to your full medical record. Please also tell us about any over-the-counter and herbal remedies you take.
- Do you take any other medications?
- Are you allergic to any medications?
- Do you have any other medical conditions?
- Have you ever had any operations?
- What's your average menstrual cycle like? How often do you get your period? How long does it last? Is it heavy or painful?
- When did your periods start? And if you've gone through the menopause, when did they stop?
- When was your last smear test?

- Have you ever been pregnant? (Including live births, terminations and pregnancy losses, e.g. miscarriages, ectopic pregnancies, stillbirths).
- Are you using any contraception?
- What are your fertility plans?
- Do you use, or have you ever used, HRT?
- Do you have any family history of any illnesses or conditions?
- Do you smoke? Do you drink alcohol?

We usually would like to examine you, with your consent. You can wear whatever you like, but it's helpful to wear something that's easy to take on and off. Many women like to wear a long skirt that they can pull up, so they don't feel like they're having to remove all their clothes. In some clinics you'll be given a hospital gown to put on. If this is the case, you can leave your bra on, and your top if it fits under the gown. Remove the bottom half of your clothing, including underwear, but if you're wearing the aforementioned long, floaty skirt you can leave this on. The gown can be worn with the opening at the back so that when you lie down the gown lies over you like a sheet.

You don't have to remove your pubic hair, but if it makes you feel more comfortable then please go ahead. It really won't get in our way. If you're having an operation, your pubic hair may need to be shaved beforehand, but not for a clinic appointment.

What does an examination involve?

Abdominal examination – We will gently feel over your entire abdomen, from just above the pubic bone to the bottom of your ribs. We are feeling for any unusual lumps or bumps and to understand where exactly you are having pain, for example. If you have any scars on your abdomen, we will ask what operation you've had. I often find scars from previous operations that my patient hasn't mentioned during our initial chat. Even if it wasn't a gynaecological operation, it's relevant to us, because it might have an impact on any surgery we may plan to perform. For example, I was planning a laparoscopy for a patient who didn't tell me she had undergone liposuction and a tummy tuck, during which the plastic surgeon had moved her belly button and created a new one. The result was so brilliant that it took me several very close looks before I asked her, 'Is that your real belly button?' I admit I felt a bit silly asking, but I'm glad I did because when she told me it wasn't, I was able to amend my plans for her surgery. I explained that I wouldn't make a cut in her belly button as I would usually do, but instead I'd enter via a cut in the upper abdomen, as there was a higher chance of damaging something inside as a result of her previous surgery, and of me damaging her beautiful new belly button. While this is an extreme example, some scars heal so well that we may not even be able to see them until you're asleep in theatre with the extra-bright surgical light shining on you – and at that point we can't wake you up and ask you which operations you've had done.

Speculum examination – This involves inserting a speculum into your vagina. It separates the vaginal walls to allow us to see your cervix. During this examination we can take a smear test if needed, or take swabs to check for infections. A speculum is made of metal or plastic and comes in a variety of sizes. If a nurse or doctor has previously had difficulty finding your cervix it is helpful for us to know this. Some women even know that they need a certain size of speculum, so we can get it right first time. Some women prefer to insert the speculum themselves – this is no problem, just let us know.

Bimanual examination – This involves inserting two fingers into your vagina while placing our other hand on your abdomen. This is a way of assessing the size, mobility and position of your uterus, as well as feeling for masses, nodules or scarring that may be signs of endometriosis.

Any of these examinations may be uncomfortable, so please let us know if you need us to stop at any time. You will usually have a chaperone present, who is generally a member of the nursing staff: there for reassurance, to help protect your dignity, help you position yourself, and help to facilitate communication between you and the doctor during the examination.

Questions to ask your gynaecologist

We usually wrap up the consultation by asking you whether you have any questions. You may like to make a list of any questions for the gynaecologist, which could include:

- What do you think is causing my symptoms?
- Do you think I need to have a scan? What are you looking for?
- Do you think I need to have a laparoscopy? What are you looking for? If you find something, will you treat it there and then?
- Do you think my fertility will be affected?
- How can I control my symptoms?
- Are there any alternatives to the treatment you are suggesting?

More specific questions related to surgery are covered on pages 271–2.

Chapter 8

What investigations or treatments might be available to me?

Blood tests

Unfortunately there are no blood tests that can identify the cause of problematic periods or diagnose any particular gynaecological conditions, but the following blood tests may be used to help understand what is going on.

Full blood count – This counts the components of the blood, including haemoglobin, white blood cells and platelets. It can be helpful to diagnose anaemia, which is a common problem for women with heavy periods (see pages 70–2).

Luteinising hormone (LH) and follicle-stimulating hormone (FSH) – These hormones are checked in tandem, usually on Day 2–5 of your menstrual cycle. They can be useful for determining whether your symptoms are related to a hormonal condition such as PCOS, hypothalamic amenorrhoea (HA) or premature menopause. These cannot be reliably tested when you are taking hormonal contraception, so you need to stop taking these before you are tested.

Progesterone – We usually talk about 'Day 21 progesterone', which is used as a marker of ovulation. If you have ovulated, your progesterone will be high on Day 21 if you have a 28-day cycle; if your cycle is not 28 days, it will be high about 7 days after ovulation and 7 days before your period. To calculate the best time to take this test, subtract 7 from the number of days of your cycle in total (e.g. 32-day cycle – 7 days = test progesterone on Day 25). If it's low, you may not be ovulating, or you may be taking the test at the wrong time.

Testosterone – There are several types of blood test to check testosterone, and this is most commonly carried out if your doctor suspects you have PCOS.

Thyroid test – Both an underactive and overactive thyroid can have an impact on your menstrual cycle, and correcting it can correct the problem.

Clotting disorders – There are many types of blood test to check for clotting disorders. Basic tests can be performed by your GP or gynaecologist, but you may be referred to a haematologist for more specialised tests.

CA-125 – This is a blood test to check levels of a glycoprotein called Carbohydrate Antigen 125 (CA-125). This can be used to help diagnose ovarian cancer and monitor a patient's response to treatment. It is non-specific, which means that raised levels do not automatically mean you have ovarian cancer, so it's used in conjunction with an ultrasound scan to assess your ovaries. It may also be raised in women with endometrial cancer (page 139) as well as non-gynaecological cancers, including breast, bowel, lung and pancreatic cancer.

This blood test is usually performed by GPs because, as you can see on pages 220–2, the symptoms of ovarian cancer are very common, and very vague. There are lots of non-cancerous gynaecological conditions that produce similar symptoms and also cause CA-125 levels to be raised, including:

- fibroids
- endometriosis
- ovarian cysts
- pregnancy
- pelvic inflammatory disease.

Non-gynaecological conditions can also cause raised CA-125 levels. These include:

- kidney failure
- liver failure
- heart failure
- tuberculosis
- pancreatitis.

Since many conditions can raise CA-125, many women with a raised level don't have ovarian cancer, although waiting for test results to come back can be incredibly anxiety-provoking. In a British study of over 50,000 women who had CA-125 tests performed at their GP surgery, 10% of those with a raised level had ovarian cancer and 12% had another type of cancer, including breast, bowel and lung cancer. This means that 78% had no form of cancer at all.[127] It's our job as doctors to ensure that the appropriate investigations are carried out to confirm whether you do or do not have cancer. If you don't, we try to determine what is causing your symptoms.

Ovarian cancer

Ovarian cancer is the sixth most common cancer in women in the UK, with about 7,500 cases diagnosed annually.

Symptoms of ovarian cancer include:

- bloating
- feeling full very quickly, or a loss of appetite
- abdominal or pelvic pain
- needing to pass urine more often or very suddenly
- changes in bowel habit

- unexplained weight loss
- new onset of IBS symptoms in women aged over 50.

If you have these symptoms, the National Institute for Health and Care Excellence (NICE) guidelines recommend performing a CA-125 blood test. If your CA-125 level is raised, an ultrasound scan should be performed.

If these tests are abnormal and/or ovarian cancer is suspected, you would be referred to your local hospital via the Two-Week Wait pathway for suspected cancers. This means you should be seen in hospital within 2 weeks of the referral.

Further tests – including a CT scan of your chest, abdomen and pelvis – would be arranged, and you may also have a biopsy performed to confirm the diagnosis. This biopsy may be taken by a radiologist, who will perform a scan to find an area of concern and take a targeted biopsy, or during a diagnostic laparoscopy (pages 100–101).

Treatment depends on where the cancer is, how fit and well you are, as well as what you want. It may involve surgery followed by chemotherapy, or chemotherapy followed by surgery and more chemotherapy, or chemotherapy alone.

Ovarian cancer care is very structured in the UK, being carried out at specific hospitals where there is a large multidisciplinary team of gynaecological cancer surgeons, oncologists who perform chemotherapy and radiotherapy, radiologists who review scans, pathologists who perform diagnoses on tissue samples, and palliative care doctors who work to manage cancer symptoms, as well as specialist nurses, dieticians and physiotherapists, all of whom are highly trained in providing top-quality care to women with gynaecological cancers.

Ovarian cancer screening

Unfortunately this doesn't yet exist because an effective method has not yet been found. A study of over 200,000 women in the UK compared no screening to screening using an annual CA-125 blood test or an annual ultrasound.[128] The results were disappointing. The blood test was able to detect cancers slightly earlier but did not save lives, whereas the annual ultrasound did neither. The search for an effective screening method continues.

Ultrasound scans

Ultrasound scans are the most simple, and the most effective, type of scan for most gynaecological conditions. They can help to diagnose a variety of conditions, including fibroids, adenomyosis, ovarian cysts, polyps and endometrial thickening. With regards to endometriosis, endometriomas can be reliably seen on an ultrasound, but it usually requires someone with very specialist skills to detect deep endometriosis. With improvements in scanning technology, some specialists may also be able to see superficial endometriosis. Your GP will often arrange an ultrasound before referring you to a gynaecologist. Unfortunately, I often see patients with terrible symptoms who have been told, 'There's nothing wrong with you because your scan looks normal', but even if your scan is normal, your symptoms are valid and a normal scan should not be the end of the road for investigating and treating your symptoms.

Not all gynaecologists perform scans themselves, but that doesn't make them bad doctors. Each doctor chooses niches during their training: some people may be very good at scanning while others don't perform complex ultrasound scans but have other skills instead. In some hospitals, you may have a scan carried out by the gynaecologist during your appointment with them, or with a sonographer (a person trained in performing scans who is not a doctor). Unfortunately, not all clinics are set up to perform a scan at the same time as your appointment.

We usually perform gynae scans internally, using a small probe inserted into the vagina. This is also known as a 'transvaginal scan'. This allows us to get closer to the organs in your pelvis. If you've never had penetrative vaginal intercourse, you can still have an internal scan. It is also possible to do an internal scan by inserting the probe into your rectum. I understand this is not something that everyone will want, but it is an option. You can also have a transabdominal scan, which means using the probe externally over your abdomen, as we do during pregnancy, although this may provide us with less information than an internal scan.

Computerised tomography and magnetic resonance imaging scans

These are rarely used for diagnosis in gynaecology, but in other specialties they are often the scan type of choice. It is not unusual to find an unexpected condition when you are scanning for something else: for example, if a woman has a CT scan to check for kidney stones, she may be found to have an ovarian cyst, or a woman having an MRI for back pain may be found to have a thickened endometrium. In these situations we may still opt to perform an ultrasound scan, because it may give us more information. CT scans can be used to investigate gynaecological cancers, and to determine whether there has been any spread of the cancer. MRI scans are most often used in endometriosis to plan surgery, and are sometimes used to further characterise ovarian cysts and to assess endometrial cancer before surgery.

Non-hormonal medication

Iron tablets – If you're anaemic, these tablets will correct this deficiency. This is discussed on pages 71–2.

Painkillers – Many people think that over-the-counter painkillers are ineffective, but they can actually be quite helpful, especially when taken regularly. However, for a lot of the conditions discussed in this book, alone they are not enough, but they can be helpful in conjunction with some of the medications and treatments mentioned below.

NSAIDs (non-steroidal anti-inflammatory drugs) such as diclofenac and ibuprofen – These reduce pain by blocking the enzyme that the body uses to produce prostaglandins, which are the chemicals involved in producing period pain. Ibuprofen appears to be the most effective NSAID[129] – more effective than paracetamol for this purpose.[130] In addition, they are able to reduce bleeding by up to 30%.[131]

Mefenamic acid – While this is an NSAID, it is prescribed specifically for painful periods and can reduce the amount and duration of bleeding by up to 50%.[132,133] It is frequently prescribed with tranexamic acid.

Paracetamol – This is an alternative for people who can't take NSAIDs. It may reduce pain in about half of women who try it.[134]

Opiates – e.g. codeine, tramadol.

Tranexamic acid – This is a very popular non-hormonal treatment for heavy bleeding that can be very effective. I frequently prescribe it for patients who come into hospital via A&E with very heavy bleeding, and I'm often surprised by how good it is at reducing bleeding very quickly, even when taken in tablet form. It reduces bleeding by acting on the blood clotting system, which may be overactive in cases of heavy bleeding. It can reduce bleeding by up to 50%,[133] and is effective in up to two-thirds of cases.[135] It can be used for sudden episodes of heavy bleeding, or on a regular basis, with some patients keeping a stock at home and taking it when their period starts. If it doesn't improve bleeding within the first two cycles it's unlikely to do so, so an alternative should be discussed. It can be used while trying to get pregnant, as it has no impact on your hormones. We also use it as an injection during surgery to reduce heavy bleeding.

Hormonal medication

Using the term 'hormonal medication' can elicit a strong reaction in many people. I speak to a lot of women who voice their distress about going to their doctor to discuss problems with their periods and being 'shoved on the pill' without much discussion. It is frustrating that we don't have more targeted treatments and medications for the gynaecological conditions discussed in this book, and that hormonal medications can have terrible side effects, but there are very valid reasons why hormonal medications are effective for many period-related issues. In some women they can be life-changing – in a positive way. I think it's important to explain this, so this section will cover how these medications work, their benefits and their side effects (which may help you to make a decision about what you might like to try). Please remember that all of these medications can be used alongside any lifestyle changes, and I actively encourage this.

Most of the hormonal medication I will discuss here is primarily designed to be used as a contraceptive, but many women take these medications for their non-contraceptive effects, which I describe to my patients as 'the good side effects' of these medications. They are commonly used for period-related problems due to their ability to thin the endometrium, which usually results in lighter – and sometimes less painful – periods. They may also make periods stop altogether, which can come as a relief for many women, although it may not suit everyone.

I speak to a lot of women who are worried about the impact of hormonal contraception on their fertility. Large studies have shown that these drugs do not damage your fertility in the long term, and this is shown by the fact that the number of women who became pregnant within a year after stopping hormonal contraception was no different when compared with women who had stopped using non-hormonal forms of contraception.[136]

However, it's important to make people aware that there may be a temporary delay in full fertility returning, depending on the type of contraception used. Here are some numbers, to give you an idea of the duration we are talking about:

Hormonal coil – 2 menstrual cycles

Contraceptive implant – 2 menstrual cycles

Contraceptive pill and vaginal ring – 3 menstrual cycles

Contraceptive patch – 4 menstrual cycles

Depot injection – 5–8 menstrual cycles.

Interestingly, users of the copper coil (which contains no hormones) also had a delay in the return of their fertility of 2 menstrual cycles.[137] Having said this, many women get pregnant immediately after they stop taking contraception, so even if you were not using it primarily for contraception, if you don't want to get pregnant please use an alternative, such as condoms, straight away.

The length of time you take hormones also has no impact on return to full fertility, so there's no need to take a break every now and then. If you feel that your body needs a break due to experiencing side effects from a specific type of hormonal contraception, that's a different matter. I'd advise you to speak to your doctor to consider changing to a different type of medication (e.g. a pill with a different strength or active ingredient, or a different method altogether), depending on why you're taking it.

Concerns regarding cancer are also common. The combined oral contraceptive pill (COCP), which is the most commonly used (and therefore the type of medication for which we have the most data) has been shown to reduce your risk of endometrial, ovarian and colorectal cancers while taking the pill – and for at least 25 years after stopping this type of medication. The COCP is, however, known to slightly increase the risk of developing cervical and breast cancers. Based on recent data, the risk of breast cancer appears to be the same whether you take the POP or COCP. (There's more information on this in the box on page 246.)

Just as with HRT, there are steps we can take to reduce our risk of breast cancer, such as ensuring we keep active and moderate our alcohol intake (discussed on pages 52–3).

This chapter also covers the negative side effects of the use of hormones. Some may be mild and manageable, but others will have such a negative impact on your quality of life that it makes them completely intolerable. Patients often ask me whether they're likely to get side effects from hormonal medication, and unfortunately there's no way to predict this. The Lowdown (www.thelowdown.com) is a very helpful website written by healthcare professionals with experience in prescribing contraception. It features reviews of all types and brands of contraception, written by users, so you can see what other people's experiences have been. Ultimately, though, everyone reacts slightly differently to medications so the only way to be sure is to try it yourself. Our hormones change as we age, so your hormonal make-up isn't going to be the same at 38 as it was at 18, for example. For this reason, you may find that a pill you loved in your early twenties doesn't suit you in the same way when you take it in your late thirties. Unfortunately, there is no way to work out which medication is going to suit you when. If someone discovers one, I'll be the first to let you know! But for now, it's a case of trial and error.

What does 'off-licence' use of a medication mean?

Drug manufacturers must obtain a licence from the Medicines and Healthcare Products Regulatory Agency (MHRA) and the European Medicines Agency (EMA) for each medication that goes onto the market. To obtain this, they must provide evidence that the medication is safe and effective to be used for a specific condition(s) at a specific dose or dosing regimen. Over time, we sometimes find that the drug is useful for other conditions besides the one specified on the licence, or that different doses are helpful, but it's very unusual for a drug manufacturer to apply for a new licence for their medication. Instead, doctors may choose to recommend use of the drug in a way that is 'off-licence' (this is also called 'off-label'). For example, the tailored methods of using the COCP (see pages 240–2) are an off-licence way of taking these tablets because they are being taken differently to the dosage described during the licensing process.

It's up to the doctor prescribing the medication to decide whether or not to do so: they need to feel comfortable enough with the available evidence to support this off-licence use, and they must be able to support their decision if you encounter problems after taking the drug. This is why your GP may not feel comfortable prescribing a medication that a gynaecologist may do, because it may be beyond the scope of their practice. This is an important point to make: all doctors need to operate within their own boundaries to provide safe healthcare, so different specialties and teams must work together to provide holistic care for patients.

The combined oral contraceptive pill (COCP)

This is the most commonly used type of contraceptive pill, and contains a synthetic oestrogen and progesterone. There are 20 COCPs currently available on the UK market, with different combinations of types and doses of oestrogen and progesterone. Most COCPs come in packets of 21 pills: you take one each day, followed by a 7-day break, then you start the next packet. A small number of pills available in the UK have 21 active pills and 7 dummy pills, which just means you take a sugar pill for seven days instead of a pill containing any active ingredients. Some women find this useful because it means they keep up the habit of taking a pill every day, so they are less likely to forget to take it or fail to start the new packet on time.

The primary mode of action through which the COCP works is by stopping the feedback link between the ovary and the brain to stop ovulation, which means that pregnancy cannot occur. The riskiest time to miss a pill (if you're using it for contraception) is at the end or the start of the pill packet (i.e. having an 8-day break instead of 7, or missing Day 2, for example), because you can get something called 'escape ovulation', where the lack of hormones for longer than designed allows your ovaries to jump back into action and pop out an egg, which could result in pregnancy. This is especially true for the modern COCPs, with their relatively low doses of hormones, that don't suppress the ovaries as strongly as the older, higher-dose versions.

The pill also has many non-contraceptive effects, due to their ability to keep the endometrium thin, as this reduces bleeding as well as pain. They can also help with symptoms related to hormonal fluctuations, due to their ability to provide a steady stream of hormones rather than the troughs and peaks seen with a natural cycle. A big advantage of the COCP over other types of hormonal contraception is that you – the user – decide whether you want to have a bleed or not and, if so, when (see pages 240–2).

While this section focuses on the COCP, combined hormonal contraception can also come in the form of a vaginal ring or patch, both of which release a synthetic oestrogen and progesterone. The NuvaRing® is made of a flexible plastic. It's worn inside the vagina for 3 weeks continuously then removed for 7 days, which is equivalent to the 7-day pill-free break with the COCP (and the time when you would usually have a bleed). The Evra® patch is applied directly to an area of hairless skin and reapplied weekly. It's worn for 3 weeks in total followed by 7 days without a patch. The patches are generally pretty robust so should stay in place during showering and exercise, but it's good practice to check it's still there afterwards. The ring and the patch provide the same non-contraceptive benefits, and come with similar side effects as the COCP: however, much of the published data concentrates on the pill because it's more widely used and has been in use for much longer.

The non-contraceptive benefits of combined hormonal contraception

Reduction in bleeding – Through its ability to reduce excessive thickening of the endometrium and stabilise it, there may be up to a 50% reduction in bleeding and the number of days of bleeding.

Reduction in period pain – This form of contraception can reduce the amount of prostaglandin produced by the endometrium, which is one of the causes of period pain. The added benefit with the COCP is that you can choose not to have a bleed by using a tailored method (see pages 240–2), thus eliminating the associated pain.

Ability to control timing of bleeding – Through the use of tailored regimes.

Endometriosis – Hormonal contraception can reduce pain and bleeding, reduce the size of endometriomas, and – when used after surgery – may reduce the risk of endometriomas recurring, reduce the chance of painful periods returning, improve sexual function and improve quality of life.

Adenomyosis – It can reduce the amount and duration of bleeding, reduce period pain and reduce the size of the uterus.

PCOS – It can be used to manage menstrual irregularity, reduce the risk of endometrial hyperplasia, and improve symptoms caused by excess androgens.

Reduction in frequency and severity of menstrual migraine.

Improvement in skin problems, including acne and hirsutism (excess hair growth).

Improvement in PMS and PMDD symptoms – The drospirenone-containing COCP is the first-line medical treatment for these conditions.

A reduction in lifetime risk of some cancers – The longer you take it, the greater the protective effect. These cancers include:

- Ovarian cancer – Women who have ever used the COCP have a 33% reduction in their risk of ovarian cancer compared to those who have never used it. This protective effect may last up to 30 years after stopping the COCP.[138] Women with mutations in the BRCA1 or BRCA2 genes, which increase their lifetime risk of ovarian cancer, will also see a protective effect.
- Endometrial cancer – Women who have ever used the COCP have a 34% reduction in their risk of endometrial cancer compared to those who have never used it. This protective effect may last up to 30 years after stopping the COCP.[138]
- Colorectal (bowel) cancers – Women who have ever used the COCP have a 19% reduction in their risk of colorectal cancer compared to those who have never used it. This protective effect may last up to 30 years after stopping the COCP.[138]

The side effects of combined hormonal contraception

This list is not exhaustive, but here are the most common and the most serious side effects that are reported.

Mood changes – It is incredibly common for women to report low mood or mood swings with use of COCP, although studies are inconclusive regarding whether these are truly caused by the COCP. There are so many confounding factors that contribute to depression and mood disorders, and it's difficult to take these into account in studies. The only way to be certain that a symptom is related to the pill is to stop it and see whether your mood improves. It is also possible to change to a different type of COCP to see if your symptoms improve, if you'd like to continue this type of medication. You might have to try a few to find the one that suits you best. Some women even report an improvement in mood. Using a tailored regime may work if the negative impact on mood is associated with the pill-free break.

Loss of libido – Sexual desire is a complex phenomenon, influenced by many external factors as well as hormones. The evidence regarding loss of libido on the pill is inconclusive, with some studies showing a decrease, some reporting no change, and others reporting an increase in libido with COCP use. However, if you find that your libido is negatively affected, it can be distressing. There appears to be a higher chance of this happening with COCPs with a lower oestrogen dose, so changing to a type with a higher dose could help.

Headaches – These are common and may improve within the first few months of use, but are a common reason for women to stop taking the COCP. If they occur or are worse during the pill-free break, using a tailored regime may help.

Nausea – This can be related to the oestrogen content of the COCP. It's usually temporary, but if it persists and is problematic you could try switching to a different COCP or try a progesterone-only medication instead. You could also try taking your pill right before bed to see if that helps.

Breast tenderness and/or enlargement – This can occur as a result of oestrogen-induced breast development and fluid retention. Just like many other symptoms, it may or may not resolve with time.

Unscheduled bleeding – This is common during the first month of use and generally improves within the first 3–4 months. If it is still happening after this time, it is important to report it to your doctor to ensure that other causes are ruled out. It is also more common with lower oestrogen doses and with specific types of progesterone, so it may be possible to change to a different pill with either a higher dose of oestrogen or a different type of progesterone, to combat the issue.

Blood clots in the arms, legs and lungs (venous thromboembolism or VTE) – This is a relatively rare complication, but it's important to be aware of it. Symptoms include a swollen, painful arm or leg which may also be red or discoloured, with prominent blood vessels. You may also experience a sudden shortness of breath and coughing up blood. The risks associated with hormonal contraception are discussed in more detail below.

Increased risk of heart attacks and strokes – These conditions are caused by clots forming in the arteries (as opposed to veins, as described above). This is a very rare occurrence in younger women, and the absolute number is also very low: an estimated two heart attacks per 100,000 women using COCP and one ischaemic stroke per 100,000 women using COCP, although these are both up to twice the rate that may be expected in the general population of women aged under 50.[139] These are serious events and must be taken seriously. For this reason, we usually avoid prescribing the COCP if you have additional risk factors for strokes and heart attacks, including high blood pressure, migraines with an aura (an aura is a warning sign that a migraine is about to happen: most commonly flashing lights or other visual disturbance), or if you are over 35 and you also smoke.

Increased risk of breast cancer – There is a small and temporary increased risk of breast cancer that disappears within 5–10 years of stopping the COCP (see the box on page 246 for further information).

Increased risk of cervical cancer – There is a small and temporary increased risk of cervical cancer that disappears within

5–10 years of stopping the COCP (see the box on pages 261-2 for further information).

Switching to a progestogen-only pill (POP) may help with some of the oestrogen-related side effects mentioned above: a recent study showed that the majority of ex-COCP users who experienced nausea, headaches, breast tenderness and swelling while on the COCP did not suffer from these on the POP.[140]

When the pill was designed and introduced back in the 1960s, the amount of oestrogen in each pill was up to ten times higher than in pills available today. This caused a lot of side effects, including bloating, breast tenderness and mood swings. The 7-day break was designed to give women relief from these side effects, and it was thought that women would see a monthly bleed as a reassuring sign that they were not pregnant. Believe it or not, I have also heard that this 7-day break was also designed to appease the Pope, who was staunchly against contraception: scientists hoped to make it more acceptable to him by making it mimic a woman's natural cycle!

Today there is good evidence that there are no health benefits to taking the 7-day break with current COCPs. Gynaecologists have long been advising women with problematic periods to take their pills 'back to back' – this means to take two or three packs in a row without a break, meaning fewer periods. This can be helpful if you have bad period pain, very heavy periods, anaemia related to your periods, PMS or headaches. This is often recommended for women with endometriosis to reduce their symptoms. The other benefit of not taking a break – or taking a short 4-day break – is that it actually makes the pill a more effective contraceptive. This is because it reduces the time that your ovaries are unsuppressed, therefore reducing the chance of ovulation.

There are several tailored regimes you can use to take your pill if you don't want to take a break and have a bleed, and these are described in Table 8.1.[141] This way of taking the pill is off-licence (see box on pages 230–31) but is heavily backed by robust scientific evidence and supported by the Faculty of Sexual and Reproductive Healthcare.[142] You must speak to your doctor before using any of these regimes, to be sure that your pill can be used on one of these tailored regimes. They can only be used with monophasic COCPs (those with the same amount of active ingredient in each tablet) containing ethinylestradiol as their active ingredient, and this doesn't apply to all COCPs on the UK market. You cannot use these regimes with the POP.

Name of regime	How you do it	Number of bleeds per year
Extended use (also known as tricycling)	3 packs in a row followed by a 4- or 7-day break	5
Flexible extended use	Minimum one pack. Maximum – as many packs as you want. You might decide to stop and have a bleed if you're getting a lot of spotting, or you just fancy having a bleed	You decide!
Continuous use	Minimum one pack. Maximum – as many packs as you want. You might decide to stop and have a bleed if you're getting a lot of spotting, or you just fancy having a bleed	Depends on your body – but possibly none!
Reduced hormone-free interval	One pack, followed by a 4-day break	15 bleeds per year

Table 8.1. *Tailored regimes for combined hormonal contraceptives.*

Studies have shown these tailored regimes do not increase the risk of endometrial hyperplasia (see page 139) or blood clots,[143] and they have no impact on future fertility.[144] The main downside to taking several packets back to back is that you could experience bloating, spotting or cramping the longer you go without taking a break.

This depends on the individual. While some women never get this, others may experience it after two packs, and some after four or five. If this happens, you can simply take a 4- or 7-day break, which will allow you to have a bleed, then start taking the pill again. As explained above, you must not take more than a 7-day break if you want to maintain the contraceptive effect. If you stop taking it for longer than 7 days, you will need another form of contraceptive, such as condoms.

How will my doctor choose a contraceptive pill for me?

There are several factors to consider, including:

- Are there any reasons why you shouldn't take the pill? This depends on whether you've ever had a blood clot, have high blood pressure, you smoke or have migraines. The POP is often more suitable if you have any of these.
- Why do you want to use the COCP or POP? Certain ingredients may be beneficial for some conditions (e.g. COCPs containing co-cyprindiol can help acne, and drospirenone can also be helpful for acne, as well as PMS and PMDD).
- Have you been on the pill before? If so, was there a pill that you did or did not like and would like to try again, or don't want to try again?

If you're on a pill containing lower oestrogen you have a higher chance of experiencing unscheduled bleeding (i.e. spotting or bleeding when you're not expecting it).[145] Most doctors will start by prescribing one of the most common COCPs containing 30 micrograms of ethinylestradiol (which is slightly higher than in many pills so carries a lower chance of unscheduled bleeding) and 150 micrograms levonorgestrel (a progesterone with the lowest associated risk of blood clots) (see box below). If you experience oestrogen-related side effects, such as nausea, bloating or breast tenderness, you could consider switching to a COCP with lower oestrogen. It's also possible to change to a COCP containing a different type of progesterone if you don't get on with the pill you have been prescribed.

If you are experiencing side effects that you find unmanageable, please speak to your doctor – they will usually be able to prescribe an alternative.

Blood clots and the contraceptive pill

Combined hormonal contraception (the COCP, contraceptive patch or vaginal ring) can slightly increase your risk of blood clots in veins. This can include deep vein thrombosis (DVT: a clot in the arm or leg) and pulmonary embolism (PE: a clot in the lung). This is because oestrogen can alter your blood's ability to clot. While it's the oestrogen in the COCP that increases the chance of clots, the exact risk seems to depend on the type of progesterone the pill contains. This is slightly confusing because progesterone alone (e.g. in the progesterone-only pill) doesn't increase your risk of clots.

I think it would be useful to share some numbers with you to put things into perspective.

Background risk of blood clots in the female population: 2 per 10,000 women:

1. Risk with COCP containing
   - Levonorgestrel, norethisterone or norgestimate: 5–7 per 10,000 women
   - Etonogestrel or norelgestromin: 6–12 per 10,000 women
   - Drospirenone, gestodene or desogestrel: 9–12 per 10,000 women
2. Risk during pregnancy: 29 per 10,000 women
3. Risk during the first 6 weeks after having a baby: 300 per 10,000 women

The risk of blood clots from combined hormonal contraception is highest in the first few months of use, which is one of the reasons that it's not recommended to start and stop these medications frequently. This means, for example, taking it for a few months, stopping for a month or two then restarting it rather than simply taking the usual 4- or 7-day pill-free break.

Having a blood clot can be dangerous: it's estimated that 1% of women who experience a blood clot from hormonal contraception may die as a result.[142] Thankfully, this is very rare, and clots are treated using blood-thinning medications.

If you want to check your pill, the active ingredients are printed on the box and on the information leaflet. Alternatively, speak to a pharmacist or the GP, doctor or nurse who prescribes your medication. This risk of clots is one of the reasons we ask about your medical history before prescribing hormonal medication. In addition, the COCP usually needs to be stopped for 4 weeks before many types of operation due to its risk of blood clots, so please always make sure you tell your doctor that you're taking the pill if you are due to have an operation, even if it's not gynae-related.

The POP, contraceptive implant and hormonal coil, along with all non-hormonal contraceptives, do not increase your risk of blood clots.

Breast cancer and hormonal contraception

While very few cases of breast cancer are related to hormonal contraception use, I believe that all women should have all the facts they need to make a decision about whether or not to take the pill. If you have a family history of cancers or any known genetic alteration, this is particularly important for you. I recommend you speak to your doctor to help you make a decision.

COCP – There may be a 20% increased risk of breast cancer during use of the combined oral contraceptive pill. This sounds like an alarmingly high number, but in real terms this equates to one extra breast cancer case diagnosed for every 7,690 women aged 15–49 using hormonal contraception for 1 year.[146] This increased risk is only seen in women who have used the COCP for 5 years or more, after they stop the pill, and disappears within 5–10 years of stopping the pill. If you have a family history of breast cancer, then you have a higher risk of breast cancer compared to the general population, but using the COCP does not further increase that risk.[142] If you have a mutation in the BRCA1 or BRCA2 gene you have a higher risk of breast and ovarian cancer. In this situation, the protective effect of the COCP on ovarian cancer risk outweighs the increased risk of breast cancer.

Progesterone-only contraceptives (POP, hormonal coil, contraceptive injection and implant) – The data examining the link between progesterone-only contraceptives and breast cancer has been inconclusive, but a recent study of women in the UK showed that use of this type of contraceptive also appears to be associated with a 20–30% increased risk of breast cancer.[147] The risk is related to the age at which you use this medication, and equates to one extra case of breast cancer per 12,500 women using progesterone-only methods aged 16–20, one extra case per 1,640 women using it aged 25–29, and one extra case per 377 women using it aged 35–39. The risk appears to decline after stopping use.

Progestogens

These are a group of progesterone-like medications that can improve bleeding symptoms, thanks to their ability to reduce excessive thickening of the endometrium, stop blood vessels from forming, reduce inflammation within the uterus lining, and reduce its production of prostaglandins (which contribute to period pain). They can be given in tablet form, as injections, implants or as an intrauterine coil. The hormonal coil and progestogen-only pill (POP) act by thickening cervical mucus to prevent sperm from travelling through the cervix to meet an egg. They also slow down the movement of the egg through the fallopian tube and keep the endometrium very thin and inactive, to reduce the chance of a pregnancy implanting in it. While the injection and implant also have the same capabilities, they act as a contraceptive by preventing ovulation. Maintaining a thin, inactive endometrium will help with bleeding. However, with all these medications there is a chance of consistent spotting or irregular bleeding patterns: this affects about 20% of users, and is a common reason to stop these medications.[1] The coil is consistently the most effective way to reduce heavy and painful bleeding, although not everyone likes the idea of having something inside their body, so the other progesterone-based therapies may be more acceptable alternatives.

Hormonal coil, e.g. Mirena®, Kyleena® and Jaydess®

The coil (Figure 8.1) is a small (about 3cm long and wide) plastic T-shaped device that is inserted through the cervix and sits in the endometrial cavity of the uterus. Strings hang from the bottom through the cervix and into the top of the vagina, and these can be used to remove the device. Hormonal coils contain the synthetic progesterone levonorgestrel, which is slowly released into the uterus. It acts by thickening cervical mucus, preventing sperm from swimming up through the cervix to meet an egg. It also causes thinning of the endometrium, so that a fertilised egg is unable to implant. The hormonal coil also prevents ovulation in about 25% of women,[148] although this is not its primary mechanism of action. Its thinning effect on the endometrium is what produces many of the non-contraceptive benefits (listed below). The amount of hormone it releases declines with time, so some women may report that their bleeding control is less effective as the device comes to the end of its life. However, it is still as effective as a contraceptive. A small amount of the active ingredient, levonorgestrel, finds its way into the bloodstream, which can result in side effects such as acne, breast tenderness and headaches, although they usually reduce in severity over time.

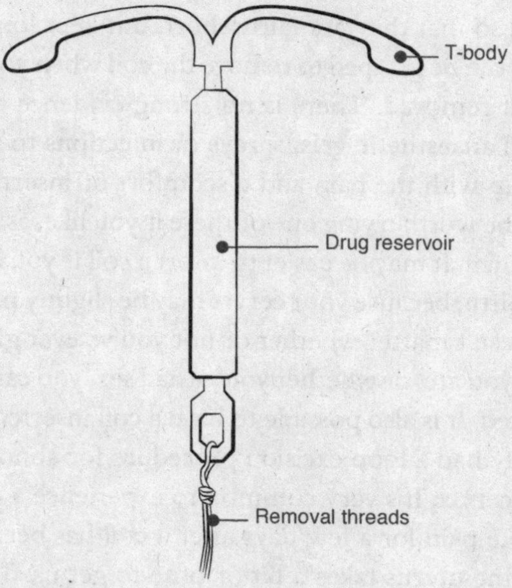

Figure 8.1. *Diagram of a hormonal coil.*

Insertion of the coil can be extremely painful for some women, while others breeze through it and barely notice. This pain, or worrying about the pain, can be a barrier to using a coil. Insertion requires a speculum examination so that the doctor or nurse inserting the coil can see your cervix. Sometimes an instrument may be used to grasp your cervix to help insertion. The coil comes in a little insertion device that looks like a drinking straw, and is used to insert the coil through the cervix and into the uterus. Once in place, the insertion device is removed and the arms of the coil spring out. The threads of the coil (which are also called strings) hang through the cervix into the top of the vagina. These are trimmed so that they are fairly short, but kept long enough that they can be grasped to remove the coil when you're ready to have it removed. There is no strong evidence to suggest that local anaesthetic gels, sprays or injections to the cervix really help with the pain and discomfort of insertion, but it may still be worth trying one of these if you like, as they don't do any harm. It may be easier to insert a coil if you have had a vaginal birth, because your cervix may be slightly more open, but it doesn't matter whether or not you've ever given birth, how old you are, or whether you've had sex, you can still have a coil fitted. It is also possible to have a coil inserted if you've previously had a loop excision procedure for abnormal cells on your cervix. It's very common to experience a cramping, period-like pain for a few days after a coil has been inserted because the uterus takes a bit of time to get used to having something inside.

There is a 3–5% chance of the coil falling out, and this is most common in the first 3 months after insertion. The risk is higher in women with fibroids and in those with heavy bleeding, and it may happen without you realising it. Given the size of the blood clots that some women pass, a tiny coil can easily go unnoticed inside one. I've often seen women in clinic who want to discuss other options to resolve their heavy bleeding because their Mirena® coil has stopped working, and when I've performed a speculum examination, then an ultrasound scan, I have realised that their coil has fallen out during a heavy period – and that's probably why they've started experiencing heavier periods.

If you are using a coil, and particularly if you have heavy bleeding, I recommend that you check your strings after each period by inserting a finger into your vagina and feeling for them, especially if you are using the coil for contraception. If you can't feel the strings, you should use condoms until it's located, and you should contact your GP, who will be able to examine you to see if the strings are visible. If they are, you're good to go! If they aren't, you'll need an ultrasound scan. Sometimes the coil is still in the correct place but the strings have become tucked up inside your cervix, but if it isn't seen on the ultrasound you will need an X-ray to check whether the coil has made a hole through the wall of the uterus and migrated up into the abdomen, which is called 'perforation'. The risk of perforation is very low (1–2 per 1,000 women), and the chance of this happening is highest if the coil is inserted when you are breastfeeding.[148] If this happens, you would need laparoscopy (keyhole surgery) to remove it. This does not usually need to be done as an emergency unless the doctor is concerned that the coil has travelled into the bowel, or a blood vessel, or you have significant pain.

Removal of a correctly positioned coil is usually very simple: a doctor or nurse will carry out a speculum examination to see the threads, which they will then grasp with an instrument and swiftly remove. Most people look at me in shock afterwards and say, 'Oh – was that it?!' And I usually – with their permission – show them the coil that I've removed as proof. Occasionally coils can be tricky to remove. If the strings are nowhere to be found, but the coil is shown to be inside the uterus on an ultrasound, it is sometimes possible to use a special coil thread retriever in clinic. This is a device that can be inserted into the uterus to try to catch the misplaced threads to remove a coil. If this is not possible, you would need a hysteroscopy to remove it. This can be done in clinic while you are awake, or in the operating theatre with sedation or a short general anaesthetic (see pages 272–3 for more about hysteroscopy). I would say that the Mirena® coil is the contraceptive that most of my colleagues in the field of O&G use for themselves, due to its convenience and its non-contraceptive benefits (listed below).

There is no lower age limit for using a coil. If one is inserted in a woman aged over 45, it can be left until she reaches the menopause or no longer needs contraception.

There are currently five types of hormonal coil on the UK market. They are:

- Mirena®, Levosert® and Benilexa® – 52mg levonorgestrel. They are licensed for use for 5 years for contraception and for heavy bleeding. Only the Mirena® is licensed for endometrial protection (it can be used for 4–5 years), but Levosert and Benilexa can be used off-licence for this purpose.
- Kyleena® – 19.5mg levonorgestrel. It is licensed for use for 5 years for contraception.
- Jaydess® – 13.5mg levonorgestrel. It is licensed for use for 3 years for contraception.

The non-contraceptive benefits of the hormonal coil

The two lower-dose hormonal coils (Kyleena® and Jaydess®) are relatively new compared to the original Mirena® 52mg version, therefore the majority of the data we have relates to the 52mg hormonal coil, which is also the only coil licensed for a use other than to provide contraception. While these lower-dose coils may have some non-contraceptive benefits, they are likely to be less than the benefits of the 52mg coil, so the benefits listed below *only apply to the 52mg coil.* They are:

Reduction in bleeding – Periods are usually much lighter, with studies reporting up to a 90% reduction in blood loss. This is usually achieved within the first 3–6 months of use.[149] After 12 months, 20% of women will have stopped having periods, and this rises to 50% after 2 years of use.[150] The coil has consistently been shown to be more effective than oral medication, including tranexamic acid, oral progestogens and the contraceptive pill, in reducing the amount of bleeding and improving quality of life. The results related to quality of life are similar to those reported after a hysterectomy.[151] It can also reduce anaemia related to heavy periods.[152] For these reasons, NICE recommends the 52mg hormonal coil as the first line of treatment for heavy bleeding.

Reduction in period pain – Studies suggest that the coil is as effective as the COCP at reducing period pain.[153] This is related to its ability to reduce inflammation and the production of prostaglandins.

Endometriosis – It reduces pain and bleeding, and can be used after surgery to reduce the risk of the disease recurring.

Adenomyosis – It is effective at reducing period pain related to adenomyosis, and over 75% of women using it for this reason would recommend it.[154] NICE recommends the 52mg hormonal coil as the first-line treatment for heavy bleeding where there is evidence of adenomyosis.

Fibroids – The coil may reduce bleeding but will not reduce the size of the fibroids. You can use a coil if your uterus is not too enlarged by the fibroids, and if you don't have a large fibroid distorting the inside of the uterus, but there is a higher chance of the coil falling out (11% fall out in women with fibroids compared to 3% in women without[53]).

PCOS – The coil reduces the risk of endometrial hyperplasia.

HRT – It can be used as the progesterone component of your HRT regime. This means you could use it alongside an oestrogen cream/gel/patch/tablet. It may be helpful to manage the erratic, heavy and painful bleeding that many women experience during the perimenopause, due to intermittent ovulation. The coil also offers contraception, which is still important during the perimenopause.

Treatment of endometrial hyperplasia – The coil has been shown to improve the chance of regression of hyperplasia, and reduce the chance of it progressing to cancer.

Reduction in risk of endometrial cancer – Through the coil's ability to reduce excessive thickening of the endometrium.

Likely reduction in risk of ovarian cancer – However, the hormonal coil is a relatively new type of medication compared to the COCP, so the data regarding this is less robust as there has been less time to study outcomes.

The side effects of the hormonal coil

Unscheduled bleeding – This can range from spotting to bleeding like your usual period and is very common, especially during the first 3 months. It usually settles with time and, as described above, bleeding may stop entirely. For some women, this remains problematic, and is the reason they have the device removed.

Mood changes – Some users report a change in mood, most commonly depressive symptoms. Some studies report a higher risk among users, while others show no association.[155] It's difficult to conclude that it is caused by the coil, but if you are concerned that your coil is affecting your mood, please talk to your GP. And remember, it can easily be removed.

Acne – Studies report that some women develop acne or, if they have acne, it worsens after the insertion of a hormonal coil, although many women report no change to their acne.[156] Interestingly, most studies do not report on the type of contraception used prior to coil insertion, so if a woman is using the COCP, which may improve acne, prior to using the coil, it isn't necessarily the coil that is associated with the acne, but stopping using the COCP. If you have acne, it is still possible to use other types of acne treatment at the same time, and you can explore this with your GP or dermatologist.

Breast tenderness – This may occur due to fluid retention and progesterone-induced development of breast tissue, although is less common using the coil than using the COCP.

Headaches – These are also less common with the hormonal coil than with the COCP, but can occur.

Increased risk of breast cancer – There is a small, temporary increased risk of breast cancer. This disappears within

5–10 years of removing the hormonal coil. (See box on pages 246–7 for further information.)

Ectopic pregnancy – This means a pregnancy that implants somewhere other than the uterus, usually in the fallopian tube (where an egg is normally fertilised). This link between ectopic pregnancy and using the hormonal coil is confusing, and causes a lot of anxiety. The contraceptive failure rate for the Mirena® coil is about 0.2% (or two pregnancies per 1,000 users). If you were unlucky enough to get pregnant with a hormonal coil in place, 25–50% of these may be ectopic pregnancies,[157] because the active ingredient of the coil reduces the mobility of the fallopian tubes, meaning a fertilised egg can get stuck there. For comparison, the rate of ectopic pregnancy in the general population is just over 1%. So while the chance is much higher with the coil, your chance of pregnancy itself is very low, therefore your overall chance of an ectopic pregnancy compared to non-coil-users is actually lower. If you get pregnant with a coil in place, you need to speak to your GP to arrange an urgent early pregnancy scan to check the location of the pregnancy. If you have severe abdominal pain, bleeding, shoulder pain, if you feel faint or collapse, you must go to A&E straight away. The increased risk of ectopic pregnancy associated with the coil goes away once you stop using it, so if you have it removed to try to get pregnant you no longer have a higher chance of ectopic pregnancy.

The progestogen-only pill (aka 'mini-pill')

The progestogen-only pill (POP), which is also known as the mini-pill, contains synthetic progesterone. The most common type of POP prescribed in the UK contains desogestrel, which causes periods to stop completely in about 20% of women.[158] There are some other POPs that contain other types of progestogen, although they are less frequently prescribed because they need to be taken within a 3-hour window to maintain their contraceptive effect, compared to the 12-hour window with desogestrel. While the POP can help with heavy periods, the COCP and hormonal coil are generally recommended before the POP because they tend to result in less unscheduled bleeding and spotting than the POP (which is why it doesn't feature in the NICE guidance for heavy bleeding). However, if there are reasons that you can't use the COCP or coil, or would prefer not to, then the POP may be a great alternative for you. They can be used from your first period up to the age of 55.

A new POP may be introduced soon, called Slynd®. It contains a progestogen called drospirenone and, unlike any other POP, is taken for 24 days with a 4-day pill-free break in the style of COCPs. During this time you may have bleeding, which is referred to as 'scheduled bleeding' because it happens within a predictable timeframe due to the pill-free break, as opposed to unscheduled bleeding, which happens at random. The benefit of this newer pill is that it can reduce the number of days of unscheduled bleeding/spotting,[159] which is great, because this is one of the most common side effects of this type of medication, and a common reason to stop using the POP. Slynd also has a slightly more forgiving 24-hour window within which you need to take it, so if you're a bit late taking your pill, it will still work as a contraceptive. Drospirenone has an anti-androgen effect, unlike most other progestogens, so this new type of POP may also be less likely to cause acne and hair loss, and may even reduce these symptoms.

The non-contraceptive benefits of the POP

Reduction in amount of bleeding – While the POP doesn't feature in the NICE guidelines for treatment of heavy periods, many users report their periods are lighter, and around 20% of women will stop having periods altogether.

Reduction in period pain – In a study of women with moderate or severe period pain, 93% reported that their pain improved or disappeared entirely within 3 months of starting the POP, and 85% said they would like to continue the medication at the end of the study.[140]

Endometriosis – Reduction in pain and bleeding symptoms.

Adenomyosis – Reduction in pain and bleeding, but no impact on size of uterus.

PCOS – A lower risk of endometrial hyperplasia, as the POP helps to maintain a thin endometrium. If you have PCOS and your periods stop on the POP, you do not need to do anything to bring on a bleed in the way you would if you were not using any hormonal medication, because with the POP the progestogen in the pill is counteracting the oestrogen that your body makes, protecting your endometrium from hyperplasia.

A possible reduction in lifetime risk of endometrial and ovarian cancers – However, this is not well proven in the literature due to the low number of women using the POP compared to the COCP.

The side effects of the POP

Unscheduled bleeding – This may be spotting or heavier bleeding, like a period. This usually reduces over time, but is a common reason to stop using the POP. A double dose of the desogestrel POP is sometimes prescribed to reduce this unscheduled bleeding.[160]

Mood changes.

Acne.

Headaches.

Worsening of PMS symptoms.

Increased risk of breast cancer – There is a small, and temporary, increased risk, which disappears within 5–10 years of stopping the POP (see box on pages 246–7).

Hormonal contraception and cervical cancer

Cervical cancer is caused by a persistent human papillomavirus (HPV) infection. Vaginal penetration helps HPV to reach the cervix. In the vast majority of cases it clears up quickly, but when it doesn't, it can cause the cells of the cervix to become abnormal, and in a small proportion of cases cancer develops. The lifetime risk of cervical cancer in the UK is 1 in 142 (0.7%).

Hormonal contraception has been associated with a higher risk of cervical cancer. The link with the COCP has been most studied. When a women stops taking the COCP, the link very quickly becomes less strong, and is very weak 10 years after last use. In a population of 20-year-old women using oral contraceptives for 10 years, the lifetime risk may be an extra 7 to 10 cases of cervical cancer per 10,000 women. However, given that cervical screening is very effective at spotting and preventing cervical cancer, for women who take the COCP and keep up to date with screening, the extra number of cases is less, at around 2 extra cases of cervical cancer per 10,000 pill users.[161] It has been suggested that this increased risk is related to different sexual behaviour by pill users rather than the pill itself: women on the COCP may have more sexual partners and more sex, both of which increase the chance of getting an HPV infection.

The available data discussing the link between hormonal contraceptives and cervical cancer was largely compiled before widespread HPV vaccination, so your risk may be even lower if you have been vaccinated.

The contraceptive injection

The most widely available injection is Depo-Provera®, which contains the progesterone medroxyprogesterone acetate. It was introduced as a treatment for endometrial and kidney cancers back in the 1960s, and was introduced as a contraceptive in the UK in the 1990s. It is injected into a muscle, usually in your bottom or upper arm, and slowly releases progesterone over a 12-week period. About 50% of users will stop having periods by the fourth injection.[162] There can be a delay in return of fertility of about 5–8 menstrual cycles,[137] which is probably because the progesterone can take some time to dissolve away completely, so it's not ideal if you want to get pregnant immediately after stopping it, and this is something to consider when planning the timing of a pregnancy. However, it has a number of non-contraceptive benefits (discussed below) and is incredibly convenient because there's nothing for you to do in between injections: you just need to remember to make your next appointment. There is also an injection called Sayana Press® which you inject yourself every 13 weeks. It contains the same active ingredient and works in the same way as Depo-Provera®. It may sound a bit scary to inject yourself, but a lot of women say it's not as bad as they thought it would be. In a study of women who tried Sayana Press®, 87% said they found the injection easy to do, 95% said it was convenient, and 94% would recommend it to others.[163] There is no time limit for how long you can use the injection, and it can be used until the age of 50.

The non-contraceptive benefits of the contraceptive injection

These are less frequently documented in the literature because the injection is used less than pills and coils, but its benefits include:

Reduction in amount of bleeding.

Reduction in period pain.

Endometriosis – Reduction in pain and bleeding.

Adenomyosis – Reduction in pain and bleeding, but no impact on size of uterus.

PCOS – Reduced risk of endometrial hyperplasia.

Fibroids – Can reduce bleeding, help fibroids to shrink and prevent them from growing.[55]

Reduction in lifetime risk of some cancers – The longer you use the injection, the greater its protective effect. These include:

- **Ovarian cancer** – Users of the contraceptive injection have a 35% lower risk.[164]
- **Endometrial cancer** – Users have an 80% reduction in the risk of endometrial cancer than women who have never used the injection.[165]

Side effects of the contraceptive injection

If you have any side effects with the injection, you have to wait for the injection to wear off for the side effects to stop – you can't stop taking it or remove it like you can with other methods.

Slight delay in return of full fertility – As above, it may take 5–8 menstrual cycles for full fertility to return.

Unscheduled bleeding – This can range from spotting to bleeding like your usual period. It's very common, and a frequently cited reason to stop using the injection. It is also common for periods to stop completely: the chance of this increases the longer you use it.

Decrease in bone mineral density – Bone mineral density (BMD) is a measure of how much calcium and other minerals you have in your bones, and can be measured by performing a DEXA scan. When you are using the injection, your body produces less natural oestrogen, which can result in a loss of BMD. Most of this happens in the first 1–2 years then it plateaus. Loss of BMD is estimated to be around 5% after 5 years of using the injection, but the good news is that BMD recovers after you stop taking the injection.[166] To put this into perspective, women can experience a 2–8% BMD loss during pregnancy and 3–5% loss during breastfeeding for 6 months or longer (and these are also temporary). BMD recovers within 12 months of the end of a pregnancy or stopping breastfeeding.[167,168] Some doctors are concerned about women using the injection before they have achieved their peak bone mineral density, and for this reason the injection is generally avoided for women under the age of 18 unless all other medications, or contraceptives, depending on the reason to use it, have been considered. The main concern about BMD loss is that it may result in a higher risk of fractures (broken bones): however, from the currently available data, it is not clear whether users do actually have a higher risk of fractures,[169] so the contraceptive and non-contraceptive benefits of the injection likely outweigh the risks. Measures to protect BMD include doing weight-bearing exercises (e.g. walking, running, playing racket sports or lifting weights), stopping smoking, and taking calcium and vitamin D supplements if your levels are low. All women should take these measures, whether they use the injection or not, because we have a higher risk of bone weakening than men. Other types of progesterone-only and combined hormonal contraception have not been proven to cause such problems with BMD.

Injection site skin reactions – These tend to be mild and disappear quickly, and are more common after using the Sayana Press® self-administered injections.

Mood changes – While some users may report a change in mood when using the injection, studies have not proven that this is caused by the injection itself. If you experience negative changes to your mood and are struggling, please speak to your doctor.

Acne.

Headaches – These are common and often a reason to stop using the injection.

Weight gain – Unlike other types of contraception, where the link with weight gain does not appear very strong, the injection has been linked with weight gain, and this is a common reason to stop using the injection. Weight gain may be more common in those who start using it aged under 18 and who have a higher starting weight.[170] If you gain over 5% of your starting body weight in the first 6 months of using the contraceptive injection, it's likely you'll continue to gain weight.

Increased risk of breast cancer – There is a small, temporary increased risk that disappears within 5–10 years of stopping the injection – see the box on pages 246–7 for further information.

Progestogen tablets, e.g. norethisterone, medroxyprogesterone acetate (MPA, brand name Provera)

These do not offer any contraceptive effect, but they can be used to decrease bleeding over the long term as an alternative to the contraceptive pill, or as a one-off treatment to quickly stop occasional episodes of heavy bleeding. Norethisterone is the most commonly prescribed. It can also be used to delay your period for a holiday or other event, as described on pages 63–4. It is broken down by the body into ethinylestradiol, which is the oestrogen component of most COCPs. It can provide some relief from perimenopausal symptoms such as bleeding. However, it slightly increases the risk of VTE (blood clots), so medroxyprogesterone acetate may be a more suitable alternative for all purposes if you have other risk factors for developing blood clots.

When norethisterone or MPA are used on a regular basis, you may be told to take it in various ways. Taking it for 21 days from Days 5–26 of your cycle has been shown to be the most effective way of reducing bleeding: this can reduce bleeding by up to 80%.[171] Taking these tablets in this manner has been shown to be almost as effective as the coil after 3 months of use. However, only 22% of women using the tablets wanted to continue the treatment at the end of the 3-month trial compared to 77% of those on the coil.[172] The reason for this was unclear; however, progestogen tablets can have more side effects, such as bloating, breast tenderness and headaches, which makes them unappealing in the long run.

If these tablets are being used to stop sudden, heavy bleeding, you can expect them to work fairly quickly: in most people, bleeding should stop within 3 days. You would then continue the tablets for 10 days in total. This is a good time to discuss more long-term measures with your GP to prevent future heavy bleeds (and look for a cause of the bleeding, if this has not already been done).

Gonadotrophin-releasing hormone analogues (GnRHa)

These are injectable medications that last for 1 to 3 months. They block receptors in the brain to suppress ovarian function, resulting in a low-oestrogen state that is referred to as a 'medically induced menopause'. Your periods will stop because you have very little oestrogen with which to thicken the endometrium – this can be helpful to build up your haemoglobin levels if you've become anaemic due to heavy bleeding. However, side effects include menopausal symptoms such as hot flushes, night sweats and bone loss, which is why these tablets cannot be used in the long term. A maximum treatment duration of 6 months is advised, and after the first 3 months of treatment it may be necessary to take some 'add-back' hormone therapy, such as tibolone, which can reduce bone density loss, hot flushes and night sweats.[173]

Endometriosis – These tablets can reduce the pain associated with endometriosis, and may be used before surgery to suppress the disease, reducing the amount of inflammation present and the blood supply to endometriosis deposits that are due to be removed.

Adenomyosis – They may be used prior to surgery to reduce the size of the uterus and to improve anaemia.

The copper coil

Throughout this book you'll often see the hormonal coil referenced as a treatment option for various period-related problems, but never the copper coil. You may be wondering why.

The copper coil is one of the most effective contraceptives out there (99.5% effective). A little-known fact is that it can be used as emergency contraception for up to 5 days after unprotected sex, and is 99.91% effective[174] – more effective than the two 'morning-after pills' available. However, the copper coil frequently makes periods heavier and more painful, especially in the first few months, and this is the most common reason for having it removed early.[175] So while it's a great contraceptive, it's unlikely to help with any bleeding or pain-related period problems. If you need to have one inserted for emergency contraception but are worried about the impact on your periods, you can have it removed after your next period.

Fibroids – They may reduce the size of fibroids by up to 50%. Unfortunately, once you stop taking them, your periods usually return within 1–2 months and the fibroids return to their previous size within 4–6 months, which is why this treatment is reserved for before surgery. It can be used before a myomectomy or a hysterectomy, because shrinking the fibroids at this point may mean the surgery can be performed via a smaller cut, may be quicker to perform, and there's less chance of the patient needing a blood transfusion if they take these tablets before a hysterectomy.[176]

PMDD – The tablets may be used to temporarily induce a menopausal state if there is any uncertainty regarding a diagnosis.

Surgical procedures

One of my favourite things about being a gynaecologist is operating. We perform many different types of operation and procedure, and these are summarised below. One of the most important things about an operation is actually the discussions we have about it beforehand. Having an operation can be scary, and we understand that patients may be very nervous, but please don't let that put you off at least having an initial discussion about surgery. This doesn't put you under any obligation to proceed.

In this section I've tried to give you an idea of how effective each procedure may be when compared to other treatments – and the possible risks. Where I've given a percentage, your surgeon may quote something different, and this may be based on their own practice or tailored to you, so please take the percentages in this book as a guide.

Questions for your surgeon

I frequently discuss surgery in clinic with my patients, and I'll try to cover most of the questions they ask below. However, the amount of information we cover in a meeting can be overwhelming, and there may be areas that aren't covered in as much detail as you'd like. Many patients are still taking in all the information they have been given, so they're not always sure what to ask.

Many teams, especially those treating endometriosis, have a specialist nurse who you may meet or be given contact details for so that you can get in touch with them after your appointment if you have further questions. This is invaluable. If the nurse doesn't know an answer to a question, they'll speak to other members of the team, including the surgeons, to find an answer. Some common questions patients ask are:

- What does the operation involve?

- How effective will it be for my symptoms?
- What are the risks and potential complications?
- What are the alternatives?
- What will happen if I do nothing?
- How long will I need to stay in hospital?
- How long is the recovery (e.g. when will I be able to go to work, the gym, etc.)?
- How long will it be until I can resume sexual activity?
- Will I need further treatment or surgery?
- Can you suggest where I can read more about this (e.g. websites, patient information leaflets)?

Hysteroscopy

This involves passing a small rigid telescope through the cervix to get a view of the endometrial cavity. This is done to investigate heavy bleeding or bleeding after menopause, or if a scan has indicated an abnormality within the uterus, such as a polyp or fibroid. During this procedure it may be possible to remove polyps or fibroids that are pushing into the uterine cavity, divide scar tissue inside the uterus (adhesions), divide a septum (a membrane of tissue that divides the cavity in two), or remove a lost coil that has migrated high up inside the uterus. A hysteroscopy is often performed in the operating theatre under general anaesthetic (GA), but can be performed in the outpatient clinic using a slightly smaller instrument than we would use in theatre. The advantage of this is that you don't need to have a GA, and we can take biopsies and remove small polyps at the same time. Unfortunately, outpatient hysteroscopy has attracted much media attention over recent years, with many women – rightfully – speaking out about experiencing excruciating pain during the procedure. I can't deny that it can be painful. Many women have described it as like severe period pain, while about 10% report no pain and around 20% report severe, intense pain.[177] If this happens to you, you must tell the medical team and the procedure can be abandoned and rearranged under a GA. Other reasons to abandon the procedure include difficulty passing the scope through the cervix or finding something that would be better removed while you're asleep, such as large or multiple polyps or fibroids.

Whether the procedure is performed while you're awake or asleep, you can expect some cramping and watery blood-stained discharge for 24–48 hours afterwards, because we fill the uterus with fluid to open it up so we can get a really good view of what's going on inside. Depending on why you're having the procedure, we may offer to insert a Mirena® coil at the same time, but we will only do this with your permission.

Endometrial ablation

This is a procedure to treat heavy periods that can be performed during a hysteroscopy. It uses a device to burn away the endometrium and stop it from thickening up. This requires the device to make direct contact with the endometrium, so it's not suitable for women with a very large endometrial cavity or fibroids that distort the shape of the cavity because the surgeon won't be able to get enough contact between the device and the surface of the endometrium to destroy it. Endometrial ablation is not recommended for anyone planning a pregnancy. In the small number of pregnancies that have occurred after ablation, there has been a higher risk of complications, including miscarriage, stillbirth and having to deliver by Caesarean section.[178] Up to 70% of women will never have periods again[179] – but if they do, they should be much lighter.

Ablation is unlikely to be effective if you have significant adenomyosis. While the procedure may result in lighter periods, the technique is only designed to remove the superficial endometrial layer; it doesn't penetrate deep enough to destroy the endometrial-like tissue deep inside the muscle layer. While periods afterwards may be lighter, many women report ongoing cyclical pain, which may even be worse than before the procedure.

While the procedure can be incredibly effective and has reduced the number of women who need to have a hysterectomy, about 20% of women who have ablation will go on to have a hysterectomy due to ongoing or recurrent symptoms. Ablation is not recommended if there is any suspicion of abnormal pre-cancerous or cancerous changes within the endometrium. A biopsy will be taken beforehand to confirm this.

Laparoscopy (aka keyhole surgery)

Laparoscopy, also known as keyhole surgery, was introduced to the field of gynaecology in the 1930s, and its use continues to increase year on year. While it can take longer for surgeons to train to perform laparoscopy compared to open surgery, it's worth the time investment for patients, who benefit from less blood loss, a shorter hospital stay and faster overall recovery. It's also quite fun to learn – I have fond memories of practising training drills such as cutting out paper circles and threading string through plastic hoops using a laparoscopy simulator balanced on an ironing board in my living room during the very early days of my surgical training.

Numerous procedures can be carried out via laparoscopy, ranging from a diagnostic laparoscopy (which is simply looking inside to investigate pelvic pain) to simple procedures such as removing ovarian cysts, to more complex operations such as treating endometriosis. These are sometimes done using robotic surgery, a type of keyhole surgery – it's still performed by a human being, but they sit at a robotic console. The main advantage of this is that the surgeon has a greater range of motion of their instruments, so it's ideal for more complex procedures.

If you're having a diagnostic laparoscopy, your pre-surgery discussion with your surgeon will cover what they might find, and what they might do about it, and this will be listed on the consent form that you'll sign before the operation. It's commonly performed to check for endometriosis. If the surgeon finds any endometriosis, they may not treat it at this initial surgery; diagnostic laparoscopy is often performed by general gynaecologists, and if you have severe disease you will need surgery carried out by an endometriosis surgeon. Or the endometriosis could involve other organs, such as the bowel, so it will need surgery with a bowel surgeon at hand. This can be very frustrating for the patient, but it's important that the right person with the right experience and support does the surgery to ensure you have the safest, most effective operation.

While the cuts made are tiny and from the outside it might not look like you've had a big operation, it's important to remember that it's still an operation and does require some recovery time. This will depend on the type of operation you've had. I've included some tips for recovery on pages 290–2.

Dye test

This is a test to check whether your fallopian tubes are open. It may be offered at the time of laparoscopy if you're having difficulty getting pregnant. It involves injecting a blue dye through the cervix to see if it spills back up and out through your fallopian tubes into your pelvic cavity. If the tubes are open, the blue dye can be seen spilling out of the tubes through the camera during keyhole surgery. If no dye is seen, this suggests the tubes are blocked. Occasionally we see the tubes dilating with the dye because of a blockage. Unfortunately, there is no successful way of unblocking the tubes, so your surgeon will discuss the next steps with you based on your individual situation. You will notice a small amount of blue dye coming out through your vagina after the operation, so it's important to wear a pad afterwards.

It's possible to check whether your fallopian tubes may be blocked without doing an operation, using a technique called hysterosalpingogram (HSG) or Hysterosalpingo Contrast Sonography (HyCoSy). Both involve placing a speculum into the vagina and passing a tube into the uterus to inject a dye that travels up through the uterus. If the fallopian tubes are open, the dye will be seen inside the tubes using X-ray (HSG) or ultrasound (HyCoSy). This procedure can also detect polyps, fibroids and scar tissue inside the uterus, which can also interfere with fertility. It's important to have swabs taken beforehand to rule out any infections that could be pushed further up inside your pelvis by the dye during the procedure. If an infection is found, it should be treated before having the procedure.

Surgery for endometriosis

Endometriosis surgery is well documented to improve quality of life.[33] This procedure is usually performed using minimal access techniques (laparoscopy or robotic surgery), because this enables the surgeon to get a very good view of the surfaces inside your abdomen and pelvic cavity. Recovery is usually quicker from a laparoscopy than from open surgery, but there are times when open surgery is necessary. It is possible to remove the endometriosis (in a process called excision surgery) or destroy it (using surgical instruments to deliver an electric current or laser; this is called ablation). Excision is generally favoured over ablation, because it is associated with a better improvement in pain symptoms.[40] This is probably because with ablation you cannot be sure whether any disease is present under the surface of the endometrium, or whether it has been destroyed. Scar tissue can be removed to detach tissues and organs that have become stuck to one another. Sometimes these may be impossible to detach, and in this case part of the bowel or bladder may have to be removed. This usually requires a stoma to be created, to drain the stool or urine respectively. Your surgeon will explain what they intend to remove prior to your surgery, and this will be detailed on the consent form that you sign. It's common for surgeons to get your permission to operate in areas that we may not need to operate in: we discuss the worst-case scenario beforehand so that we can do what needs to be done during the surgery.

It is common for women to need repeat surgery due to recurrence of symptoms.[33] After surgery, your surgeon will talk to you about hormonal medications to reduce the risk of symptoms or the disease recurring.

Hysterectomy

This is an operation to remove the uterus, usually including the cervix, with or without removing the ovaries (this is called an oophorectomy). It is common to remove the fallopian tubes at the same time, because they have no function apart from transporting eggs into the uterus, and this isn't needed once the uterus is removed – and because removing the tubes can reduce your risk of ovarian cancer, even if your ovaries are left behind. Removal of the fallopian tubes is called a salpingectomy. Removal of both the tubes and ovaries is called a salpingo-oophorectomy – quite a mouthful!

I've often heard women say they've had a 'partial hysterectomy'. This isn't really a thing, so here's a run-down of the types of hysterectomy you can have (Figure 8.2):

Total hysterectomy – This is the most common type of hysterectomy. It means removal of the uterus, including the cervix and tubes. It can be performed using any of the techniques below. The cervix is disconnected from the top of the vagina, which is then sutured closed at the top, so the entire vagina will remain.

Subtotal hysterectomy – This involves removal of the uterus and tubes, but means that your cervix remains in place. In this situation you'll need to keep having cervical screening tests for cervical cancer, so it's important to clarify with your surgeon whether your cervix has been removed or not.

Radical hysterectomy – This is usually only performed if a patient has cervical cancer. It involves removal of the parametrium (the tissue next to the uterus) and the top one-third of the vagina as well as the uterus, cervix and fallopian tubes (with or without the ovaries). While your vagina will be slightly shorter after this procedure, it will still be possible for you to have penetrative sex once you've healed.

Your surgeon will discuss whether to remove your ovaries or leave them in place. This decision depends on several factors, including the reason for the hysterectomy, whether you've gone through the menopause, whether you have any known genetic risk factors, and – of course – your wishes. If your ovaries are removed, you will go into a surgical menopause (see box on pages 283–4).

If your ovaries are left in place they will still function, so you won't go into menopause. Many women still have a hormonal cycle and can, for example, experience premenstrual symptoms such as bloating and mood changes, but without periods. Eggs will also be released each month. These will be absorbed by your body without causing any problems.

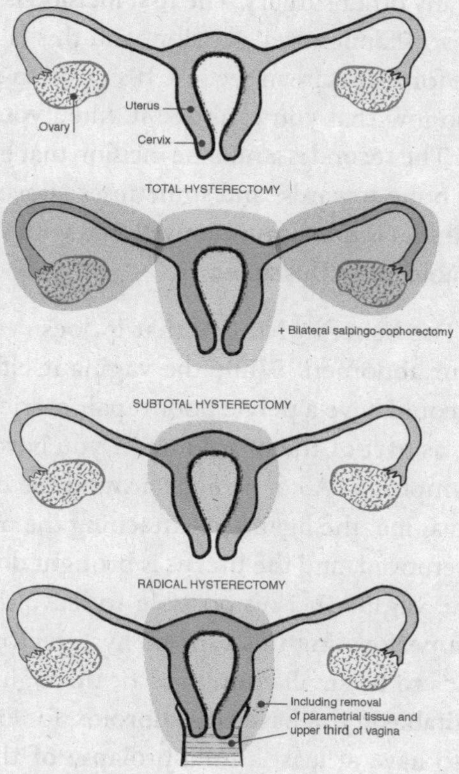

Figure 8.2. *Types of hysterectomy.*

There are also several ways to perform a hysterectomy:

Open/abdominal – This is the most traditional way of performing a hysterectomy. There are two types of surgical incision, the size and location of which depends on factors including the size of your uterus, whether the surgeon is concerned that it's stuck to any other organs, and whether you've had any other surgery. The first incision is called a low transverse or 'Pfannenstiel' incision, and this is the incision that's made for a Caesarean section. It's a side-to-side cut that is usually so low that you can't see it when you're wearing underwear. The second is a midline incision that goes up from your pubic bone towards, and sometimes above, your belly button. The skin is most commonly closed with stitches, usually dissolvable, or with staples.

Vaginal – The benefit of this is that it doesn't require any cuts on your abdomen. While the vagina itself remains in place, you could have a pelvic floor repair carried out at the same time, as part of the procedure, if you have significant prolapse symptoms. A cut is made around the cervix at the top of the vagina, the ligaments attaching the uterus to the pelvis are removed, and the uterus is brought down and out through the vagina. It isn't possible to leave the cervix in place when performing this type of hysterectomy, and the uterus needs to be small enough to fit through the vagina, so it's unsuitable if you have large fibroids, for example. You also need to have at least a mild prolapse of the uterus to do this, because otherwise the uterus is held up too tightly by the ligaments inside the pelvis, making the operation almost impossible.

Laparoscopic (aka keyhole) – The main benefits of a keyhole procedure are that you will have several small cuts rather than one large cut, less risk of heavy bleeding during the surgery, a shorter hospital stay and an overall faster recovery. The uterus is detached from its blood supply and the ligaments that hold it up, a cut made around the top of the vagina, the uterus is removed through the vagina, and the top of the vagina closed with stitches. Alternatively, a small cut can be made low down in the abdomen to remove the uterus if it won't fit through the vagina.

Robotic – As discussed on pages 275–6.

Surgical menopause

- Surgical menopause will start immediately after both ovaries have been removed. Your symptoms will be more sudden, and possibly more severe, than those experienced by women going into a natural menopause.
- Whether you want to use hormone replacement therapy (HRT) and when to start it will depend on your circumstances and wishes, and should be discussed before surgery.

- If you have had a hysterectomy along with the removal of your ovaries, you'll only need oestrogen, which can be given as a tablet, cream/gel or patch, rather than oestrogen with progesterone, as the progesterone component is used as a safety measure for women with a uterus, because unopposed oestrogen (i.e. without progesterone) could otherwise cause a dangerous overgrowth of the endometrium. Since you don't have a uterus, this is no longer a problem.
- If you still have a uterus, you'll need combined oestrogen/progesterone HRT to protect your endometrium.
- If you have endometriosis, the British Menopause Society suggests the use of a combined oestrogen/progesterone HRT, even if your uterus has been removed, as oestrogen-only HRT may cause the growth of any remaining endometriotic deposits. Tibolone is another option in this scenario.[180]
- Removal of a single ovary will not cause surgical menopause, but your natural menopause may come about 1–2 years earlier than it would normally do.[181]
- Removal of both fallopian tubes, either with or without hysterectomy, induces a surgical menopause. It does not appear to hasten the start of the natural menopause.[182]

Myomectomy

This is an operation to remove fibroids and can be carried out in several ways, depending on the size and location of the fibroids. A myomectomy can be really helpful to relieve the pressure symptoms, reduce bleeding, and increase your chance of pregnancy if the fibroids are pressing into the uterine cavity. While every case is individual, performing a myomectomy is often more complicated, time-consuming and less effective in the long term than performing a hysterectomy. Myomectomy is used as a fertility-sparing surgery for women who plan to get pregnant afterwards – or who would like the option. If you are certain that your family is complete, a hysterectomy may be more suitable for you, because after large fibroids are removed, any tiny fibroids that remain may start to grow into a much larger fibroid, which could leave you back in the same situation you started in. Regrowth is more common the younger you are. Just under 25% of women who have a myomectomy will require further surgery within 5 years.[183]

Here are the different techniques for a myomectomy:

Hysteroscopic – Also known as TCRF (TransCervical Resection of Fibroid). This is only suitable for fibroids that are pressing into the endometrial cavity. A hysteroscopy is performed at the start of the procedure to check the location of the fibroids – and that they are amenable to being cut out using this technique. A resectoscope is then passed through the cervix. This is a slightly larger telescope with a semi-circular loop of wire through which an electric current is passed: this is used to shave the fibroid away. The shavings are removed from the uterus at the end of the procedure. If the fibroid is particularly large, you may be offered GnRH analogues to shrink it in the weeks leading up to the surgery, and it may be necessary to perform a two-step procedure, with a second operation to complete the removal.

Open abdominal – This is ideal for fibroids that are pushing out of the uterus. A surgical incision will be made (either from side to side or up and down, depending on the size of the fibroid(s), a cut will be made on the uterus, through which the fibroids are taken out, and the uterus will be stitched back up. I particularly enjoy laying the fibroids out in size order after the operation to take photos to show my patients, who are usually fascinated. I often end up removing more fibroids than the scans suggest, because during the procedure we often find smaller fibroids that are hidden on the scan by larger fibroids. Please ask your surgeon beforehand if you would like to see photos: we don't routinely do this, but it's an extra service that I like to offer!

Laparoscopic or robotic – This may be an alternative to open myomectomy, depending on the size and location of the fibroids. Your surgeon will discuss this with you based on the scans performed prior to the operation. The cuts are very small, around 1cm long, so you may be wondering how the fibroids will be removed. The answer is through morcellation: this means that they are cut into small pieces, to allow them to be removed more easily. Due to the tiny risk of fibroids being cancerous, which increases with age (pages 119–20), morcellation is not recommended if you are over 50 years old. It is also possible to place the fibroid(s) in a bag inside your abdomen then morcellate them, to contain the tiny pieces in one place. They are then removed bit by bit, along with the bag, at the end of the operation. This part can be incredibly time-consuming but the benefit to the patient (a quicker recovery) makes it worth the effort. There is no evidence that one method is better than the other in the long term with regards to risk of recurrence.[184] As with any type of keyhole surgery, there is a risk that the surgeon will need to convert to an open procedure if there are any problems during the surgery: the chance of this may be up to 10%. Both open and keyhole myomectomy carry a 2–4% chance of having to convert to a hysterectomy if there is very heavy bleeding that cannot be controlled by other means.[185]

Myomectomy during a Caesarean section – While this sounds like a great idea (two operations in one!) it is best avoided, due to the significant risk of heavy bleeding due to the phenomenal blood supply of a pregnant uterus. The only time I've removed a fibroid during a C-section was because the location of the fibroid made the uterus impossible to close once the baby had been born.

Your surgeon will discuss with you the ideal length of time to wait after surgery before trying to conceive, if this is what you want. A general figure is about 6 months. The surgeon will also discuss their recommendations for the type of birth you should have. While some women may be advised to have a Caesarean section (based on factors including the size and location of fibroids removed), many women will be able to have a vaginal birth.

Uterine artery embolisation (UAE)

This is a procedure performed by a radiologist rather than a gynaecologist. It involves passing a small tube through the femoral artery in your groin, tracing it along to the uterine artery that supplies your uterus, then injecting a substance that blocks off the artery, resulting in shrinkage of fibroids and a decrease in bleeding, while preserving your uterus. You don't need to have a GA to have UAE done. You may also hear it referred to as uterine fibroid embolisation. You'll usually need to stay overnight in hospital. It can be very painful afterwards because the fibroids are essentially dying off, so you'll receive strong painkillers and sometimes a patient-controlled analgesia pump (a drip containing morphine or similar painkillers that you can safely self-administer by pressing a button). Post-embolisation syndrome is a common, flu-like illness that can develop after the procedure as your body mounts an inflammatory response to the death of the fibroids. It can last up to 2 weeks.

Vaginal discharge after this procedure is very common and can go on for several months. Some women report passing pieces of fibroid, most commonly after UAE for submucous fibroids.

UAE is generally more effective for smaller fibroids. It may be unsuitable for pedunculated fibroids that (if subserosal) could fall off into the abdominal cavity, or (if submucous) could fall off into the uterine cavity and get stuck in the cervix.

There is a chance that you may go into the menopause after UAE, if particles intended to block the blood supply to the fibroid travel away and block the blood supply to your ovaries. The chance of this happening is higher if you are over the age of 45.[186]

UAE is very effective at shrinking fibroids and reducing bleeding symptoms, although it appears less effective for symptom control than myomectomy or hysterectomy.[187] It does mean that women can avoid surgery and a general anaesthetic (although around 30% of women who have UAE will go on to have either myomectomy or hysterectomy within 5 years of their UAE).[188]

Pregnancy is possible after UAE, although there is little data to confirm the safety of this – you will need to discuss this with your gynaecologist if UAE is your preferred treatment option. Pregnancy rates are lower and miscarriage rates higher following UAE than in women who have had a myomectomy.[189]

More recently, UAE has also been used for women with adenomyosis. The results appear promising; again, there is very little data to suggest that pregnancy is safe afterwards.

Magnetic resonance-guided focused ultrasound (MRgFUS)

This is another non-surgical procedure that shrinks fibroids while leaving your uterus in place. It's also performed by radiology doctors, although it's not currently available in NHS hospitals. It uses MRI and ultrasound to focus heat energy onto your fibroids to destroy them, and can reduce bleeding symptoms and the size of fibroids.

It's generally avoided if you also have adenomyosis, have very large or multiple fibroids, or if your bladder or bowel sit in front of the fibroids (as they may be damaged by passing ultrasound waves during the procedure).

Top tips for recovering from open abdominal or keyhole surgery

- Wear soft, stretchy underwear and clothing to go home from hospital and for the next few weeks – you don't want anything that's going to dig in or rub on your stitches, plus you may feel quite bloated, especially if you've had keyhole surgery, because we inflate your abdomen with CO_2 gas so that we can see all your organs.
- Take a pillow or folded towel to put across your abdomen in the car on the way home – this will stop the seatbelt from digging in, and some women find that applying pressure over the pillow/towel helps when going over bumps. This is a great hack that I learned from my patients – it really helped me after I had my Caesarean section.
- Don't get constipated. This is unpleasant at the best of times, but when you've got a sore abdomen from surgery, no thanks! Drink lots of fluids, eat plenty of fibre, and consider taking a mild laxative, especially if you're taking painkillers that make you prone to constipation, such as codeine.
- Keep hydrated. As well as reducing your chance of constipation, keeping hydrated reduces your risk of

blood clots. Lots of people also report having a dry mouth after an anaesthetic, so keep sipping!

- Eat chewing gum and drink coffee. Both help to stimulate your bowel, which can be sluggish after surgery.
- Drink mint tea. This may help with bloating and the gassy pain that you can get in your stomach and shoulders after keyhole surgery.
- Wear stockings. You'll be given thrombo-embolus deterrent (TED) stockings to wear in hospital. I recommend wearing these at home until you're back to your usual mobility – to reduce the risk of blood clots, as they're primarily intended, but also to reduce puffiness, which is quite common after surgery and can be uncomfortable.
- Stay mobile. This helps to reduce the risk of blood clots, reduces swelling, reduces the risk of constipation, and can also help with general healing.
- Rest. Even if you have a tiny external scar that you can barely see, you've still had surgery inside. Allow your body time to heal. If you like to sleep on your front, propping yourself up with pillows or using a pregnancy pillow can help to get you into a nice position to sleep, as you'll probably find it too uncomfortable to sleep on your stomach at first.

Conclusion

The scope of gynaecological problems is huge, and can be overwhelming. I hope that you have found the topics covered in this book useful and educational. There is A LOT more that I wanted to write about, but there just wasn't enough space. There is a list of resources at the end of this book that I think will be helpful if you want to learn more about a certain topic. However, a book can only do so much: if you are – or if someone close to you is – experiencing problems with your periods or wider gynae health, I hope that this book acts as a prompt for you to seek the medical attention that you deserve.

I also want to take this opportunity to say 'thank you' to the thousands of patients who have shared their experiences with me, allowing me to gain an insight into what having gynaecological problems is like. Hearing your stories is incredibly humbling, and seeing how women still manage to get through the day despite pain and discomfort, demonstrates how strong we really are. And in the moments where you don't feel strong, please remember that there is someone out there who cares, who wants to listen to you and help you.

While there are no specific, targeted treatments for many of the conditions listed in this book, there are a lot of treatments that can help. You are never alone. Having health issues can feel very isolating, especially when it comes to gynaecological health, because many women feel like they should keep quiet about these topics. I can tell you with a reasonable degree of certainty that you probably know someone who has experienced the same thing as you are, so I encourage you to be brave and speak out. You're likely to find support closer to home than you expect.

Notes

1 Critchley HOD, Babayev E, Bulun SE, et al. 'Menstruation: science and society.' *Am. J. Obstet. Gynecol.*, 2020, 223(5): 624–64. doi:10.1016/j.ajog.2020.06.004
2 Macklon NS, Geraedts JP, Fauser BC. 'Conception to ongoing pregnancy: the "black box" of early pregnancy loss.' *Hum. Reprod. Update*, 2002, 8(4): 333–43.
3 Johnson S, Marriott L, Zinaman M. 'Can apps and calendar methods predict ovulation with accuracy?' *Curr. Med. Res. Opin.*, 2018, 1–18. doi:10.1080/03007995.2018.1475348
4 Fraser IS, McCarron G, Markham R, et al. 'Blood and total fluid content of menstrual discharge.' *Obstet. Gynecol.*, 1985, 65(2): 194–8.
5 Moore J, Barlow D, Jewell D, et al. 'Do gastrointestinal symptoms vary with the menstrual cycle?' *Br. J. Obstet. Gynaecol.*, 1998, 105(12): 1322–5. doi:10.1111/j.1471-0528.1998.tb10014.x
6 McClintock MK. 'Menstrual synchrony and suppression.' *Nature*, 1971, 229(5282): 244–5. doi:10.1038/229244a0
7 O'Herlihy C, Robinson HP, de Crespigny LJ. 'Mittelschmerz is a preovulatory symptom.' *Br. Med. J.*, 1980, 280(6219): 986. doi:10.1136/bmj.280.6219.986
8 Dasharathy SS, Mumford SL, Pollack AZ, et al. 'Menstrual bleeding patterns among regularly menstruating women.' *Am. J. Epidemiol.*, 2012, 175(6): 536–45. doi:10.1093/aje/kwr356

9 Christensen KY, Maisonet M, Rubin C, et al. 'Progression through puberty in girls enrolled in a contemporary British cohort.' *J. Adolesc. Health*, 2010, 47(3): 282–9. doi:10.1016/j.jadohealth.2010.02.005

10 Rees M. 'Menarche when and why?' *Lancet*, 1993, 342(8884): 1375–6. doi:10.1016/0140-6736(93)92746-g

11 Morris DH, Jones ME, Schoemaker MJ, et al. 'Determinants of age at menarche in the UK: analyses from the Breakthrough Generations Study.' *Br. J. Cancer*, 2010, 103(11): 1760–4. doi:10.1038/sj.bjc.6605978

12 Mishra GD, Pandeya N, Dobson AJ, et al. 'Early menarche, nulliparity and the risk for premature and early natural menopause.' *Hum. Reprod.*, 2017, 32(3): 679–86. doi:10.1093/humrep/dew350

13 National Institute for Health and Care Excellence. *Clinical Knowledge Summary: Amenorrhoea*. February 2022. Available at: https://cks.nice.org.uk/topics/amenorrhoea/

14 McKinlay SM, Brambilla DJ, Posner JG. 'The normal menopause transition.' *Maturitas*, 2008, 61(1–2): 4–16. doi:10.1016/j.maturitas.2008.09.005

15 Women's Health Concern/British Menopause Society. 'Understanding the risks of breast cancer: A comparison of lifestyle risk factors versus Hormone Replacement Therapy (HRT) treatment.' 2023. Available at: https://thebms.org.uk/wp-content/uploads/2023/01/WHC-Infographics-JANUARY-2023-BreastCancerRisks.pdf

16 Action Aid. 'Cost of living: 12% of British women are affected by period poverty.' 27 May 2022. Available at: https://www.actionaid.org.uk/blog/2022/05/27/cost-living-12-british-women-are-affected-period-poverty

17 Bowman N, Thwaites A. 'Menstrual cup and risk of IUD expulsion – a systematic review.' *Contracept. Reprod. Med.*, 2023, 8(1): 15. doi:10.1186/s40834-022-00203-x

18 van Eijk AM, Zulaika G, Lenchner M, et al. 'Menstrual cup use, leakage, acceptability, safety, and availability: a systematic review and meta-analysis.' *Lancet Public Health*, 2019, 4(8): e376–93. doi:10.1016/S2468-2667(19)30111-2

19 Meaddough EL, Olive DL, Gallup P, et al. 'Sexual activity, orgasm and tampon use are associated with a decreased risk for endometriosis.' *Gynecol. Obstet. Invest.*, 2002, 54(2): 61–2. doi:10.1159/000068354

20 El Soufi H, El Soufi Y, Al-Nuaimi S, et al. 'Toxic shock syndrome associated with menstrual cup use.' *IDCases*, 2021, 25: e01171. doi:10.1016/j.idcr.2021.e01171
21 National Institute for Health and Care Excellence. *Anaemia - Iron deficiency: How common is it?* April 2023. Available at: https://cks.nice.org.uk/topics/anaemia-iron-deficiency/background-information/prevalence/
22 Percy L, Mansour D. 'Iron deficiency and iron-deficiency anaemia in women's health.' *The Obstetrician & Gynaecologist*, 2017, 19: 155–61. doi:10.1111/tog.12368
23 Lundstrom V, Green K. 'Endogenous levels of prostaglandin F2alpha and its main metabolites in plasma and endometrium of normal and dysmenorrheic women.' *Am. J. Obstet. Gynecol.*, 1978, 130(6): 640–6. doi:10.1016/0002-9378(78)90320-4
24 Shapley M, Jordan K, Croft PR. 'An epidemiological survey of symptoms of menstrual loss in the community.' *Br. J. Gen. Pract.*, 2004, 54(502): 359–63.
25 Shapley M, Jordan J, Croft PR. 'A systematic review of postcoital bleeding and risk of cervical cancer.' *Br. J. Gen. Pract.*, 2006, 56(527): 453–60.
26 Pennant ME, Mehta R, Moody P, et al. 'Premenopausal abnormal uterine bleeding and risk of endometrial cancer.' *BJOG*, 2017, 124(3): 404–11. doi:10.1111/1471-0528.14385
27 Faculty of Sexual and Reproductive Health. *FSRH Clinical Guideline: Contraception After Pregnancy*, 2020. Available at: https://www.fsrh.org/standards-and-guidance/documents/contraception-after-pregnancy-guideline-january-2017/
28 Hirsch M, Dhillon-Smith R, Cutner AS, et al. 'The prevalence of endometriosis in adolescents with pelvic pain: A systematic review.' *J. Pediatr. Adolesc. Gynecol.*, 2020, 33(6): 623–30. doi:10.1016/j.jpag.2020.07.011
29 All Party Parlimentary Group on Endometriosis. *Endometriosis in the UK: Time for change.* Inquiry Report 2020. Available at: https://www.endometriosis-uk.org/sites/default/files/files/Endometriosis%20APPG%20Report%20Oct%202020.pdf
30 National Institute for Health and Care Excellence. *Endometriosis: Diagnosis and management*. NICE guideline [NG73]. 2017. Available at: https://www.nice.org.uk/guidance/ng73
31 ESHRE. *Endometriosis. Guideline of European Society of Human Reproduction*

and Embryology. 2022. Available at: https://www.eshre.eu/Guideline/Endometriosis

32 Bevan G. 'Endometriosis: Thousands share devastating impact of condition.' BBC, 6 October 2019. Available at: https://www.bbc.co.uk/news/health-49897873

33 Carrillo Torres P, Martinez-Zamora MA, Ros C, et al. 'Clinical and sonographic impact of oral contraception in patients with deep endometriosis and adenomyosis at 2 years of follow-up.' *Sci. Rep.*, 2023, 13(1): 2066. doi:10.1038/s41598-023-29227-2

34 Vercellini P, de Matteis S, Somigliana E, et al. 'Long-term adjuvant therapy for the prevention of postoperative endometrioma recurrence: A systematic review and meta-analysis.' *Acta Obstet. Gynecol. Scand.*, 2013, 92(1): 8–16. doi:10.1111/j.1600-0412.2012.01470.x

35 Zorbas KA, Economopoulos KP, Vlahos NF. 'Continuous versus cyclic oral contraceptives for the treatment of endometriosis: A systematic review.' *Arch. Gynecol. Obstet.*, 2015, 292(1): 37–43. doi:10.1007/s00404-015-3641-1

36 Vercellini P, Buggio L, Berlanda N, et al. 'Estrogen-progestins and progestins for the management of endometriosis.' *Fertil. Steril.*, 2016, 106(7): 1552–71e2. doi:10.1016/j.fertnstert.2016.10.022

37 Lockhat FB, Emembolu JO, Konje JC. 'The efficacy, side-effects and continuation rates in women with symptomatic endometriosis undergoing treatment with an intra-uterine administered progestogen (levonorgestrel): A 3-year follow-up.' *Hum. Reprod.*, 2005, 20(3): 789–93. doi:10.1093/humrep/deh650

38 Lockhat FB, Emembolu JE, Konje JC. 'Serum and peritoneal fluid levels of levonorgestrel in women with endometriosis who were treated with an intrauterine contraceptive device containing levonorgestrel.' *Fertil. Steril.*, 2005, 83(2): 398–404. doi:10.1016/j.fertnstert.2004.07.961

39 Kim HY, Song SY, Jung SH, et al. 'Long-term efficacy and safety of levonorgestrel-releasing intrauterine system as a maintenance treatment for endometriosis.' *Medicine (Baltimore)*, 2022, 101(10):e 29023. doi:10.1097/MD.0000000000029023

40 Pundir J, Omanwa K, Kovoor E, et al. 'Laparoscopic excision versus ablation for endometriosis-associated pain: An updated systematic review and meta-analysis.' *J. Minim. Invasive Gynecol.*, 2017, 24(5): 747–56. doi:10.1016/j.jmig.2017.04.008

41 Vercellini P, Crosignani PG, Abbiati A, et al. 'The effect of surgery for symptomatic endometriosis: The other side of the story.' *Hum. Reprod. Update*, 2009, 15(2): 177–88. doi:10.1093/humupd/dmn062
42 Opoien HK, Fedorcsak P, Byholm T, et al. 'Complete surgical removal of minimal and mild endometriosis improves outcome of subsequent IVF/ICSI treatment.' *Reprod. Biomed. Online*, 2011, 23(3): 389–95. doi:10.1016/j.rbmo.2011.06.002
43 Bafort C, Beebeejaun Y, Tomassetti C, et al. 'Laparoscopic surgery for endometriosis.' *Cochrane Database Syst. Rev.*, 2020, 10(10): CD011031. doi:10.1002/14651858.CD011031.pub3
44 Genc M, Genc B, Cengiz H. 'Adenomyosis and accompanying gynecological pathologies.' *Arch. Gynecol. Obstet.*, 2015, 291(4): 877–81. doi:10.1007/s00404-014-3498-8
45 Peric H, Fraser IS. 'The symptomatology of adenomyosis.' *Best Pract. Res. Clin. Obstet. Gynaecol.*, 2006, 20(4): 547–55. doi:10.1016/j.bpobgyn.2006.01.006
46 Naftalin J, Hoo W, Pateman K, et al. 'How common is adenomyosis? A prospective study of prevalence using transvaginal ultrasound in a gynaecology clinic.' *Hum. Reprod.*, 2012, 27(12): 3432–9. doi:10.1093/humrep/des332
47 Shaaban OM, Ali MK, Sabra AM, et al. 'Levonorgestrel-releasing intrauterine system versus a low-dose combined oral contraceptive for treatment of adenomyotic uteri: a randomized clinical trial.' *Contraception*, 2015, 92(4): 301–7. doi:10.1016/j.contraception.2015.05.015
48 National Institute for Health and Care Excellence. *Uterine artery embolisation for treating adenomyosis.* Interventional procedures guidance [IPG473]. 16 December 2013. Available at: https://www.nice.org.uk/guidance/ipg473/chapter/4-Efficacy
49 Divakar H. 'Asymptomatic uterine fibroids.' *Best Pract. Res. Clin. Obstet. Gynaecol.*, 2008, 22(4): 643–54. doi:10.1016/j.bpobgyn.2008.01.007
50 Wise LA, Laughlin-Tommaso SK. 'Epidemiology of uterine fibroids: From menarche to menopause.' *Clin. Obstet. Gynecol.*, 2016, 59(1): 2–24. doi:10.1097/GRF.0000000000000164
51 Macmillan Cancer Support. *Leiomyosarcoma.* 2022. Available at: https://www.macmillan.org.uk/cancer-information-and-support/soft-tissue-sarcoma/leiomyosarcoma

52 Mao J, Pfeifer S, Zheng XE, et al. 'Population-based estimates of the prevalence of uterine sarcoma among patients with leiomyomata undergoing surgical treatment.' *JAMA Surg.*, 2015, 150(4): 368–70. doi:10.1001/jamasurg.2014.3518

53 Zapata LB, Whiteman MK, Tepper NK, et al. 'Intrauterine device use among women with uterine fibroids: A systematic review.' *Contraception*, 2010, 82(1): 41–55. doi:10.1016/j.contraception.2010.02.011

54 Machado RB, de Souza IM, Beltrame A, et al. 'The levonorgestrel-releasing intrauterine system: Its effect on the number of hysterectomies performed in perimenopausal women with uterine fibroids.' *Gynecol. Endocrinol.*, 2013, 29(5): 492–5. doi:10.3109/09513590.2013.769517

55 Harmon QE, Patchel SA, Zhao S, et al. 'Depot medroxyprogesterone acetate use and the development and progression of uterine leiomyoma.' *Obstet. Gynecol.*, 2022, 139(5): 797–807. doi:10.1097/AOG.0000000000004745

56 Casini ML, Rossi F, Agostini R, et al. 'Effects of the position of fibroids on fertility.' *Gynecol. Endocrinol.*, 2006, 22(2): 106–09.

57 Lee HJ, Norwitz ER, Shaw J. 'Contemporary management of fibroids in pregnancy.' *Rev. Obstet. Gynecol.*, 2010, 3(1): 20–7.

58 Klatsky PC, Tran ND, Caughey AB, et al. 'Fibroids and reproductive outcomes: A systematic literature review from conception to delivery.' *Am. J. Obstet. Gynecol.*, 2008, 198(4): 357–66. doi:10.1016/j.ajog.2007.12.039

59 Bozdag G, Mumusoglu S, Zengin D, et al. 'The prevalence and phenotypic features of polycystic ovary syndrome: A systematic review and meta-analysis.' *Hum. Reprod.*, 2016, 31(12): 2841–55. doi:10.1093/humrep/dew218

60 Roos N, Kieler H, Sahlin L, et al. 'Risk of adverse pregnancy outcomes in women with polycystic ovary syndrome: Population-based cohort study.' *BMJ*, 2011, 343: d6309. doi:10.1136/bmj.d6309

61 Johnson JE, Daley D, Tarta C, et al. 'Risk of endometrial cancer in patients with polycystic ovarian syndrome: A meta-analysis.' *Oncol. Lett.*, 2023, 25(4): 168. doi:10.3892/ol.2023.13754

62 Motta AB. 'The role of obesity in the development of polycystic ovary syndrome.' *Curr. Pharm. Des.*, 2012, 18(17): 2482–91. doi:10.2174/13816128112092482

63 Toosy S, Sodi R, Pappachan JM. 'Lean polycystic ovary syndrome

(PCOS): An evidence-based practical approach.' *J. Diabetes Metab. Disord.*, 2018, 17(2): 277–85. doi:10.1007/s40200-018-0371-5

64 Minooee S, Ramezani Tehrani F, Rahmati M, et al. 'Prediction of age at menopause in women with polycystic ovary syndrome.' *Climacteric*, 2018, 21(1): 29–34. doi:10.1080/13697137.2017.1392501

65 Teede H, Deeks A, Moran L. 'Polycystic ovary syndrome: A complex condition with psychological, reproductive and metabolic manifestations that impacts on health across the lifespan.' *BMC Med.*, 2010, 8:41. doi:10.1186/1741-7015-8-41

66 ESHRE. *International evidence-based guideline for the assessment and management of polycystic ovary syndrome 2023*. Available at: https://www.eshre.eu/Guidelines-and-Legal/Guidelines/Polycystic-Ovary-Syndrome

67 Shai I, Schwarzfuchs D, Henkin Y, et al. 'Weight loss with a low-carbohydrate, Mediterranean, or low-fat diet.' *N. Engl. J. Med.*, 2008, 359(3): 229–41. doi:10.1056/NEJMoa0708681

68 Woodward A, Klonizakis M, Broom D. 'Exercise and polycystic ovary syndrome.' *Adv. Exp. Med. Biol.*, 2020, 1228: 123–36. doi:10.1007/978-981-15-1792-1_8

69 Almenning I, Rieber-Mohn A, Lundgren KM, et al. 'Effects of high-intensity interval training and strength training on metabolic, cardiovascular and hormonal outcomes in women with polycystic ovary syndrome: A pilot study.' *PLoS One*, 2015, 10(9): e0138793. doi:10.1371/journal.pone.0138793

70 NHS. *Physical activity guidelines for adults aged 19 to 64*. August 2021. Available at: https://www.nhs.uk/live-well/exercise/exercise-guidelines/physical-activity-guidelines-for-adults-aged-19-to-64/

71 Greff D, Juhasz AE, Vancsa S, et al. 'Inositol is an effective and safe treatment in polycystic ovary syndrome: A systematic review and meta-analysis of randomized controlled trials.' *Reprod. Biol. Endocrinol.*, 2023, 21(1): 10. doi:10.1186/s12958-023-01055-z

72 Menichini D, Facchinetti F. 'Effects of vitamin D supplementation in women with polycystic ovary syndrome: A review.' *Gynecol. Endocrinol.*, 2020, 36(1): 1–5. doi:10.1080/09513590.2019.1625881

73 Burkman RT, Jr. 'The role of oral contraceptives in the treatment of hyperandrogenic disorders.' *Am. J. Med.*, 1995, 98(1A): 130S–36S. doi:10.1016/s0002-9343(99)80071-0

74 Lee SC, Kaunitz AM, Sanchez-Ramos L, et al. 'The oncogenic potential of endometrial polyps: A systematic review and meta-analysis.' *Obstet. Gynecol.*, 2010, 116(5): 1197–205. doi:10.1097/AOG.0b013e3181f74864

75 Stamatellos I, Stamatopoulos P, Bontis J. 'The role of hysteroscopy in the current management of the cervical polyps.' *Arch. Gynecol. Obstet.*, 2007, 276(4): 299–303. doi:10.1007/s00404-007-0417-2

76 Nelson AL, Papa RR, Ritchie JJ. 'Asymptomatic cervical polyps: Can we just let them be?' *Women's Health*, 2015, 11(2): 121–6. doi:10.2217/whe.14.86

77 Hassa H, Tekin B, Senses T, et al. 'Are the site, diameter, and number of endometrial polyps related with symptomatology?' *Am. J. Obstet. Gynecol.*, 2006, 194(3): 718–21. doi:10.1016/j.ajog.2005.08.060

78 Nathani F, Clark TJ. 'Uterine polypectomy in the management of abnormal uterine bleeding: A systematic review.' *J. Minim. Invasive Gynecol.*, 2006, 13(4): 260–8. doi:10.1016/j.jmig.2006.03.015

79 Wang Y, Yang M, Huang X, et al. 'Prevention of benign endometrial polyp recurrence using a Levonorgestrel-releasing intrauterine system in premenopausal patients: A retrospective cohort study.' *J Minim. Invasive Gynecol.*, 2020, Sep–Oct, 27(6): 1281–6. doi:10.1016/j.jmig.2019.11.023

80 Cancer Research UK. *Uterine cancer statistics.* Available at: https://www.cancerresearchuk.org/health-professional/cancer-statistics/statistics-by-cancer-type/uterine-cancer

81 Schmid D, Behrens G, Keimling M, et al. 'A systematic review and meta-analysis of physical activity and endometrial cancer risk.' *Eur. J. Epidemiol.*, 2015, 30(5): 397–412. doi:10.1007/s10654-015-0017-6

82 Ryan NAJ, Glaire MA, Blake D, et al. 'The proportion of endometrial cancers associated with Lynch syndrome: A systematic review of the literature and meta-analysis.' *Genet. Med.*, 2019, 21(10): 2167–80. doi:10.1038/s41436-019-0536-8

83 Royal College of Obstetricians and Gynaecologists and the British Society for Gynaecological Endoscopy. *Management of Endometrial Hyperplasia (Green-top Guideline No. 67).* RCOG/BSGE Joint Guideline, February 2016. Available at: https://www.rcog.org.uk/guidance/browse-all-guidance/green-top-guidelines/management-of-endometrial-hyperplasia-green-top-guideline-no-67/

84 Mittermeier T, Farrant C, Wise MR. 'Levonorgestrel-releasing intrauterine system for endometrial hyperplasia.' *Cochrane Database Syst. Rev.*, 2020, 9(9): CD012658. doi:10.1002/14651858.CD012658.pub2

85 Gallos ID, Yap J, Rajkhowa M, et al. 'Regression, relapse, and live birth rates with fertility-sparing therapy for endometrial cancer and atypical complex endometrial hyperplasia: A systematic review and meta-analysis.' *Am. J. Obstet. Gynecol.*, 2012, 207(4): 266 e1–12. doi:10.1016/j.ajog.2012.08.011

86 Berga SL, Marcus MD, Loucks TL, et al. 'Recovery of ovarian activity in women with functional hypothalamic amenorrhea who were treated with cognitive behavior therapy.' *Fertil. Steril.*, 2003, 80(4): 976–81. doi:10.1016/s0015-0282(03)01124-5

87 NHS Digital. *NHS Maternity Statistics, England – 2021–22*. 29 November 2022. Available at: https://digital.nhs.uk/data-and-information/publications/statistical/nhs-maternity-statistics/2021-22

88 Tsuji S, Nobuta Y, Hanada T, et al. 'Prevalence, definition, and etiology of cesarean scar defect and treatment of cesarean scar disorder: A narrative review.' *Reprod. Med. Biol.*, 2023, 22(1): e12532. doi:10.1002/rmb2.12532

89 Antila-Langsjo RM, Maenpaa JU, Huhtala HS, et al. 'Cesarean scar defect: A prospective study on risk factors.' *Am. J. Obstet. Gynecol.*, 2018, 219(5): 458 e1–58e8. doi:10.1016/j.ajog.2018.09.004

90 Vissers J, Hehenkamp W, Lambalk CB, et al. 'Post-Caesarean section niche-related impaired fertility: Hypothetical mechanisms.' *Hum. Reprod.*, 2020, 35(7): 1484–94. doi:10.1093/humrep/deaa094

91 Jordans IPM, de Leeuw RA, Stegwee SI, et al. 'Sonographic examination of uterine niche in non-pregnant women: A modified Delphi procedure.' *Ultrasound Obstet. Gynecol.*, 2019, 53(1): 107–15. doi:10.1002/uog.19049

92 Florio P, Gubbini G, Marra E, et al. 'A retrospective case-control study comparing hysteroscopic resection versus hormonal modulation in treating menstrual disorders due to isthmocele.' *Gynecol. Endocrinol.*, 2011, 27(6): 434–8. doi:10.3109/09513590.2010.495431

93 Zhang J, Zhu C, Yan L, et al. 'Comparing levonorgestrel intrauterine system with hysteroscopic niche resection in women with postmenstrual spotting related to a niche in the uterine cesarean scar: A randomized, open-label, controlled trial.' *Am. J. Obstet. Gynecol.*, 2023, 228(6): 712 e1–12 e16. doi:10.1016/j.ajog.2023.03.020

94 Vervoort A, Vissers J, Hehenkamp W, et al. 'The effect of laparoscopic resection of large niches in the uterine caesarean scar on symptoms, ultrasound findings and quality of life: A prospective cohort study.' *BJOG*, 2018, 125(3): 317–25. doi:10.1111/1471-0528.14822

95 Vitale SG, Ludwin A, Vilos GA, et al. 'From hysteroscopy to laparo-endoscopic surgery: What is the best surgical approach for symptomatic isthmocele? A systematic review and meta-analysis.' *Arch. Gynecol. Obstet.*, 2020, 301(1): 33–52. doi:10.1007/s00404-020-05438-0

96 Shankar M, Lee CA, Sabin CA, et al. 'von Willebrand disease in women with menorrhagia: A systematic review.' *BJOG*, 2004, 111(7): 734–40. doi:10.1111/j.1471-0528.2004.00176.x

97 Curry N, Bowles L, Clark TJ, et al. 'Gynaecological management of women with inherited bleeding disorders. A UK Haemophilia Centres Doctors' Organisation Guideline.' *Haemophilia*, 2022, 28(6): 917–37. doi:10.1111/hae.14643

98 Collaborative Group on Hormonal Factors in Breast Cancer. 'Menarche, menopause, and breast cancer risk: Individual participant meta-analysis, including 118,964 women with breast cancer from 117 epidemiological studies.' *Lancet Oncol.*, 2012, 13(11): 1141–51. doi:10.1016/S1470-2045(12)70425-4

99 Dos Santos CCM, Uggioni MLR, Colonetti T, et al. 'Hyaluronic acid in postmenopause vaginal atrophy: A systematic review.' *J. Sex. Med.*, 2021, 18(1): 156–66. doi:10.1016/j.jsxm.2020.10.016

100 Xi D, Chen B, Tao H, et al. 'The risk of depressive and anxiety symptoms in women with premature ovarian insufficiency: A systematic review and meta-analysis.' *Arch. Women's Mental Health*, 2023, 26(1): 1–10. doi:10.1007/s00737-022-01289-7

101 Ye M, Shou M, Zhang J, et al. 'Efficacy of cognitive therapy and behavior therapy for menopausal symptoms: A systematic review and meta-analysis.' *Psychol. Med.*, 2022, 52(3): 433–45. doi:10.1017/S0033291721005407

102 Mishell DR, Jr. 'Premenstrual disorders: Epidemiology and disease burden.' *Am. J. Manag. Care*, 2005, 11(16 Suppl.): S473–9.

103 Halbreich U, Borenstein J, Pearlstein T, et al. 'The prevalence, impairment, impact, and burden of premenstrual dysphoric disorder (PMS/PMDD).' *Psychoneuroendocrinology*, 2003, 28 (Suppl. 3): 1–23. doi:10.1016/s0306-4530(03)00098-2

104 Sander B, Gordon JL. 'Premenstrual mood symptoms in the perimenopause.' *Curr. Psychiatry Rep.*, 2021, 23(11): 73. doi:10.1007/s11920-021-01285-1
105 American Psychiatric Association, DSM-5 Task Force. *Diagnostic and Statistical Manual of Mental Disorders: DSM-5™* (5th ed.). 2013, American Psychiatric Publishing, Inc.
106 Siminiuc R, Turcanu D. 'Impact of nutritional diet therapy on premenstrual syndrome.' *Front. Nutr.*, 2023, 10: 1079417. doi:10.3389/fnut.2023.1079417
107 Beddig T, Reinhard I, Kuehner C. 'Stress, mood, and cortisol during daily life in women with premenstrual dysphoric disorder (PMDD).' *Psychoneuroendocrinology*, 2019, 109: 104372. doi:10.1016/j.psyneuen.2019.104372
108 Mohebbi Dehnavi Z, Jafarnejad F, Sadeghi Goghary S. 'The effect of 8 weeks aerobic exercise on severity of physical symptoms of premenstrual syndrome: A clinical trial study.' *BMC Women's Health*, 2018, 18(1): 80. doi:10.1186/s12905-018-0565-5
109 Marjoribanks J, Brown J, O'Brien PM, et al. 'Selective serotonin reuptake inhibitors for premenstrual syndrome.' *Cochrane Database Syst. Rev.*, 2013, 2013(6): CD001396. doi:10.1002/14651858.CD001396.pub3
110 Hunter MS, Ussher JM, Browne SJ, et al. 'A randomized comparison of psychological (cognitive behavior therapy), medical (fluoxetine) and combined treatment for women with premenstrual dysphoric disorder.' *J. Psychosom. Obstet. Gynaecol.*, 2002, 23(3): 193–9. doi:10.3109/01674820209074672
111 Lopez LM, Kaptein AA, Helmerhorst FM. 'Oral contraceptives containing drospirenone for premenstrual syndrome.' *Cochrane Database Syst. Rev.*, 2012, 2: CD006586. doi:10.1002/14651858.CD006586.pub4
112 Schoep ME, Adang EMM, Maas JWM, et al. 'Productivity loss due to menstruation-related symptoms: A nationwide cross-sectional survey among 32,748 women.' *BMJ Open*, 2019, 9(6): e026186. doi:10.1136/bmjopen-2018-026186
113 Mitchell KR, Geary R, Graham CA, et al. 'Painful sex (dyspareunia) in women: Prevalence and associated factors in a British population probability survey.' *BJOG*, 2017, 124(11): 1689–97. doi:10.1111/1471-0528.14518

114 Bodyform UK. *Full period sex survey results.* 2019. Available at: https://www.bodyform.co.uk/break-taboos/our-world/full-period-sex-survey-results/
115 Qi X, Zhang W, Ge M, et al. 'Relationship between dairy products intake and risk of endometriosis: A systematic review and dose-response meta-analysis.' *Front. Nutr.*, 2021, 8: 701860. doi:10.3389/fnut.2021.701860
116 Chavarro JE, Rich-Edwards JW, Rosner B, et al. 'A prospective study of dairy foods intake and anovulatory infertility.' *Hum. Reprod.*, 2007, 22(5): 1340–7. doi:10.1093/humrep/dem019
117 LaRosa CL, Quach KA, Koons K, et al. 'Consumption of dairy in teenagers with and without acne.' *J. Am. Acad. Dermatol.*, 2016, 75(2): 318–22. doi:10.1016/j.jaad.2016.04.030
118 Uzuner C, Mak J, El-Assaad F, et al. 'The bidirectional relationship between endometriosis and microbiome.' *Front. Endocrinol. (Lausanne)*, 2023, 14: 111.
119 Korczynska L, Zeber-Lubecka N, Zgliczynska M, et al. 'The role of microbiota in the pathophysiology of uterine fibroids – a systematic review.' *Front. Cell. Infect. Microbiol.*, 2023, 13: 1177366. doi:10.3389/fcimb.2023.1177366
120 Sun Y, Gao S, Ye C, et al. 'Gut microbiota dysbiosis in polycystic ovary syndrome: Mechanisms of progression and clinical applications.' *Front. Cell. Infect. Microbiol.*, 2023, 13: 1142041. doi:10.3389/fcimb.2023.1142041
121 Nabeh OA. 'New insights on the impact of gut microbiota on premenstrual disorders. Will probiotics solve this mystery?' *Life Sci.*, 2023, 321: 121606. doi:10.1016/j.lfs.2023.121606
122 Chen P, Wang K, Zhuang M, et al. 'An insight into gut microbiota and metabolites in the mice with adenomyosis.' *Front. Cell. Infect. Microbiol.*, 2023, 13: 1075387. doi:10.3389/fcimb.2023.1075387
123 Stephansson O, Falconer H, Ludvigsson JF. 'Risk of endometriosis in 11,000 women with celiac disease.' *Hum. Reprod.*, 2011, 26(10): 2896–901. doi:10.1093/humrep/der263
124 Jehan S, Auguste E, Hussain M, et al. 'Sleep and premenstrual syndrome.' *J. Sleep Med. Disord.*, 2016, 3(5): 1061.
125 Pattanittum P, Kunyanone N, Brown J, et al. 'Dietary supplements for dysmenorrhoea.' *Cochrane Database Syst. Rev.*, 2016 3(3): CD002124. doi:10.1002/14651858.CD002124.pub2

126 Arik MI, Kiloatar H, Aslan B, et al. 'The effect of TENS for pain relief in women with primary dysmenorrhea: A systematic review and meta-analysis.' *Explore (NY)*, 2022, 18(1): 108–13. doi:10.1016/j.explore.2020.08.005

127 Funston G, Hamilton W, Abel G, et al. 'The diagnostic performance of CA125 for the detection of ovarian and non-ovarian cancer in primary care: A population-based cohort study.' *PLoS Med.*, 2020, 17(10): e1003295. doi:10.1371/journal.pmed.1003295

128 Menon U, Gentry-Maharaj A, Burnell M, et al. 'Ovarian cancer population screening and mortality after long-term follow-up in the UK Collaborative Trial of Ovarian Cancer Screening (UKCTOCS): A randomised controlled trial.' *Lancet*, 2021, 397(10290): 2182–93. doi:10.1016/S0140-6736(21)00731-5

129 Nie W, Xu P, Hao C, et al. 'Efficacy and safety of over-the-counter analgesics for primary dysmenorrhea: A network meta-analysis.' *Medicine (Baltimore)*, 2020, 99(19): e19881. doi:10.1097/MD.0000000000019881

130 Marjoribanks J, Ayeleke RO, Farquhar C, et al. 'Nonsteroidal anti-inflammatory drugs for dysmenorrhoea.' *Cochrane Database Syst. Rev.*, 2015, 2015(7): CD001751. doi:10.1002/14651858.CD001751.pub3

131 Bofill Rodriguez M, Lethaby A, Farquhar C. 'Non-steroidal anti-inflammatory drugs for heavy menstrual bleeding.' *Cochrane Database Syst. Rev.*, 2019, 9(9): CD000400. doi:10.1002/14651858.CD000400.pub4

132 Grover V, Usha R, Gupta U, et al. 'Management of cyclical menorrhagia with prostaglandin synthetase inhibitor.' *Asia Oceania J. Obstet. Gynaecol.*, 1990, 16(3): 255–9. doi:10.1111/j.1447-0756.1990.tb00235.x

133 Matteson KA, Rahn DD, Wheeler TL 2nd, et al. 'Nonsurgical management of heavy menstrual bleeding: A systematic review.' *Obstet. Gynecol.*, 2013, 121(3): 632–43. doi:10.1097/AOG.0b013e3182839e0e

134 Armour M, Parry K, Al-Dabbas MA, et al. 'Self-care strategies and sources of knowledge on menstruation in 12,526 young women with dysmenorrhea: A systematic review and meta-analysis.' *PLoS One*, 2019, 14(7): e0220103. doi:10.1371/journal.pone.0220103

135 Bryant-Smith AC, Lethaby A, Farquhar C, et al. 'Antifibrinolytics for heavy menstrual bleeding.' *Cochrane Database Syst. Rev.*, 2018, 4(4): CD000249. doi:10.1002/14651858.CD000249.pub2

136 Girum T, Wasie A. 'Return of fertility after discontinuation of contra-

ception: A systematic review and meta-analysis.' *Contracept. Reprod. Med.*, 2018, 3: 9. doi:10.1186/s40834-018-0064-y
137 Yland JJ, Bresnick KA, Hatch EE, et al. 'Pregravid contraceptive use and fecundability: Prospective cohort study.' *BMJ*, 2020, 371: m3966. doi:10.1136/bmj.m3966
138 Iversen L, Sivasubramaniam S, Lee AJ, et al. 'Lifetime cancer risk and combined oral contraceptives: The Royal College of General Practitioners' Oral Contraception Study.' *Am. J. Obstet. Gynecol.*, 2017, 216(6): 580 e1–80 e9. doi:10.1016/j.ajog.2017.02.002
139 Lidegaard O, Lokkegaard E, Jensen A, et al. 'Thrombotic stroke and myocardial infarction with hormonal contraception.' *N. Engl. J. Med.*, 2012, 366(24): 2257–66. doi:10.1056/NEJMoa1111840
140 Ahrendt HJ, Karckt U, Pichl T, et al. 'The effects of an oestrogen-free, desogestrel-containing oral contraceptive in women with cyclical symptoms: Results from two studies on oestrogen-related symptoms and dysmenorrhoea.' *Eur. J. Contracept. Reprod. Health Care*, 2007, 12(4): 354–61. doi:10.1080/13625180701536771
141 Nash Z, Thwaites A, Davies M. 'Tailored regimens for combined hormonal contraceptives.' *BMJ*, 2020, 368: m200. doi:10.1136/bmj.m200
142 Faculty of Sexual and Reproductive Healthcare. *FSRH Clinical Guideline: Combined Hormonal Contraception (January 2019, amended July 2023).* Available at: https://www.fsrh.org/standards-and-guidance/documents/combined-hormonal-contraception/
143 Hee L, Kettner LO, Vejtorp M. 'Continuous use of oral contraceptives: An overview of effects and side-effects.' *Acta Obstet. Gynecol. Scand.*, 2013, 92(2): 125–36. doi:10.1111/aogs.12036
144 Barnhart KT, Schreiber CA. 'Return to fertility following discontinuation of oral contraceptives.' *Fertil. Steril.*, 2009, 91(3): 659–63. doi:10.1016/j.fertnstert.2009.01.003
145 Gallo MF, Nanda K, Grimes DA, et al. '20 µg versus >20 µg estrogen combined oral contraceptives for contraception.' *Cochrane Database Syst. Rev.*, 2013, 2013(8): CD003989. doi:10.1002/14651858.CD003989.pub5
146 Mørch LS, Skovlund CW, Hannaford PC, et al. 'Contemporary hormonal contraception and the risk of breast cancer.' *N. Engl. J. Med.*, 2017, 377(23): 2228–39. doi:10.1056/NEJMoa1700732
147 Fitzpatrick D, Pirie K, Reeves G, et al. 'Combined and progestagen-only

hormonal contraceptives and breast cancer risk: A UK nested case-control study and meta-analysis.' *PLoS Med.*, 2023, 20(3): e1004188. doi:10.1371/journal.pmed.1004188

148 Faculty of Sexual and Reproductive Healthcare. *FSRH Clinical Guideline: Intrauterine Contraception (March 2023, amended July 2023)*. Available at: https://www.fsrh.org/documents/ceuguidanceintrauterinecontraception/

149 Dhamangaonkar PC, Anuradha K, Saxena A. 'Levonorgestrel intrauterine system (Mirena): An emerging tool for conservative treatment of abnormal uterine bleeding.' *J. Midlife Health*, 2015, 6(1): 26–30. doi:10.4103/0976-7800.153615

150 Hidalgo M, Bahamondes L, Perrotti M, et al. 'Bleeding patterns and clinical performance of the levonorgestrel-releasing intrauterine system (Mirena) up to two years.' *Contraception*, 2002, 65(2): 129–32.

151 Bofill Rodriguez M, Lethaby A, Jordan V. 'Progestogen-releasing intrauterine systems for heavy menstrual bleeding.' *Cochrane Database Syst. Rev.*, 2020, 6(6): CD002126. doi:10.1002/14651858.CD002126.pub4

152 Monteiro I, Bahamondes L, Diaz J, et al. 'Therapeutic use of levonorgestrel-releasing intrauterine system in women with menorrhagia: A pilot study.[1]' *Contraception*, 2002, 65(5): 325–8. doi:10.1016/s0010-7824(02)00283-4

153 Lindh I, Milsom I. 'The influence of intrauterine contraception on the prevalence and severity of dysmenorrhea: A longitudinal population study.' *Hum. Reprod.*, 2013, 28(7): 1953–60. doi:10.1093/humrep/det101

154 Sheng J, Zhang WY, Zhang JP, et al. 'The LNG-IUS study on adenomyosis: A 3-year follow-up study on the efficacy and side effects of the use of levonorgestrel intrauterine system for the treatment of dysmenorrhea associated with adenomyosis.' *Contraception*, 2009, 79(3): 189–93. doi:10.1016/j.contraception.2008.11.004

155 Elsayed M, Dardeer KT, Khehra N, et al. 'The potential association between psychiatric symptoms and the use of levonorgestrel intrauterine devices (LNG-IUDs): A systematic review.' *World J. Biol. Psychiatry*, 2023, 24(6): 457–75. doi:10.1080/15622975.2022.2145354

156 Barbieri JS, Mitra N, Margolis DJ, et al. 'Influence of contraception class on incidence and severity of acne vulgaris.' *Obstet. Gynecol.*, 2020, 135(6): 1306–12. doi:10.1097/AOG.0000000000003880

157 Barnhart KT. 'Clinical practice. Ectopic pregnancy.' *N. Engl. J. Med.*, 2009, 361(4): 379–87. doi:10.1056/NEJMcp0810384

158 Benagiano G, Primiero FM. 'Seventy-five microgram desogestrel minipill, a new perspective in estrogen-free contraception.' *Ann. NY Acad. Sci.*, 2003, 997: 163–73. doi:10.1196/annals.1290.019
159 Kubba A, Gemzell-Danielsson K, Palacios S, et al. 'The drospirenone (DRSP)-only pill: Clinical implications in the daily use.' *Eur. J. Contracept. Reprod. Health Care*, 2023, 28(1): 36–43. doi:10.1080/13625187.2022.21641 86
160 Burton RC, Williams CE. 'Double-dose desogestrel: Is it effective in adolescent menstrual dysfunction?' *J. Pediatr. Adolesc. Gynecol.*, 2021, 34(5): 662–65. doi:10.1016/j.jpag.2021.04.015
161 Sasieni P. 'Cervical cancer prevention and hormonal contraception.' *Lancet*, 2007, 370(9599): 1591–2. doi:10.1016/S0140-6736(07)61667-5
162 Hubacher D, Lopez L, Steiner MJ, et al. 'Menstrual pattern changes from levonorgestrel subdermal implants and DMPA: Systematic review and evidence-based comparisons.' *Contraception*, 2009, 80(2): 113–8. doi:10.1016/j.contraception.2009.02.008
163 Prabhakaran S, Sweet A. 'Self-administration of subcutaneous depot medroxyprogesterone acetate for contraception: Feasibility and acceptability.' *Contraception*, 2012, 85(5): 453–7. doi:10.1016/j.contraception.2011.09.015
164 Phung MT, Lee AW, Wu AH, et al. 'Depot-medroxyprogesterone acetate use is associated with decreased risk of ovarian cancer: The mounting evidence of a protective role of progestins.' *Cancer Epidemiol. Biomarkers Prev.*, 2021, 30(5): 927–35. doi:10.1158/1055-9965.EPI-20-1355
165 'Depot-medroxyprogesterone acetate (DMPA) and risk of endometrial cancer. The WHO Collaborative Study of Neoplasia and Steroid Contraceptives.' *Int. J. Cancer*, 1991, 49(2): 186–90.
166 Kaunitz AM, Miller PD, Rice VM, et al. 'Bone mineral density in women aged 25–35 years receiving depot medroxyprogesterone acetate: Recovery following discontinuation.' *Contraception*, 2006, 74(2): 90–9. doi:10.1016/j.contraception.2006.03.010
167 Karlsson C, Obrant KJ, Karlsson M. 'Pregnancy and lactation confer reversible bone loss in humans.' *Osteoporos. Int.*, 2001, 12(10): 828–34. doi:10.1007/s001980170033
168 Sowers M, Corton G, Shapiro B, et al. 'Changes in bone density with lactation.' *JAMA*, 1993, 269(24): 3130–5.

169 Lopez LM, Grimes DA, Schulz KF, et al. 'Steroidal contraceptives: Effect on bone fractures in women.' *Cochrane Database Syst. Rev.*, 2014, (6): CD006033. doi:10.1002/14651858.CD006033.pub5

170 Beksinska ME, Smit JA, Kleinschmidt I, et al. 'Prospective study of weight change in new adolescent users of DMPA, NET-EN, COCs, nonusers and discontinuers of hormonal contraception.' *Contraception*, 2010, 81(1): 30–4. doi:10.1016/j.contraception.2009.07.007

171 Bofill Rodriguez M, Lethaby A, Low C, et al. 'Cyclical progestogens for heavy menstrual bleeding.' *Cochrane Database Syst. Rev.*, 2019, 8(8): CD001016. doi:10.1002/14651858.CD001016.pub3

172 Irvine GA, Campbell-Brown MB, Lumsden MA, et al. 'Randomised comparative trial of the levonorgestrel intrauterine system and norethisterone for treatment of idiopathic menorrhagia.' *Br. J. Obstet. Gynaecol.*, 1998, 105(6): 592–8. doi:10.1111/j.1471-0528.1998.tb10172.x

173 Moroni RM, Martins WP, Ferriani RA, et al. 'Add-back therapy with GnRH analogues for uterine fibroids.' *Cochrane Database Syst. Rev.*, 2015, 2015(3): CD010854. doi:10.1002/14651858.CD010854.pub2

174 Cleland K, Zhu H, Goldstuck N, et al. 'The efficacy of intrauterine devices for emergency contraception: A systematic review of 35 years of experience.' *Hum. Reprod.*, 2012, 27(7): 1994–2000. doi:10.1093/humrep/des140

175 Hubacher D, Chen PL, Park S. 'Side effects from the copper IUD: Do they decrease over time?' *Contraception*, 2009, 79(5): 356–62. doi:10.1016/j.contraception.2008.11.012

176 Lethaby A, Puscasiu L, Vollenhoven B. 'Preoperative medical therapy before surgery for uterine fibroids.' *Cochrane Database Syst. Rev.*, 2017, 11(11): CD000547. doi:10.1002/14651858.CD000547.pub2

177 Harrison R, Kuteesa W, Kapila A, et al. 'Pain-free day surgery? Evaluating pain and pain assessment during hysteroscopy.' *Br. J. Anaesth.*, 2020, 125(6): e468–e70. doi:10.1016/j.bja.2020.08.015

178 Ibiebele I, Nippita TA, Baber R, et al. 'A study of pregnancy after endometrial ablation using linked population data.' *Acta Obstet. Gynecol. Scand.*, 2021, 100(2): 286–93. doi:10.1111/aogs.14002

179 Kumar V, Chodankar R, Gupta JK. 'Endometrial ablation for heavy menstrual bleeding.' *Women's Health (London)*, 2016, 12(1): 45–52. doi:10.2217/whe.15.86

180 Garg A, Robinson L. 'Surgical menopause: A toolkit for healthcare professionals.' *Post Reprod. Health*, 2021, 27(4): 222–5. doi:10.1177/20533691211038455
181 Bjelland EK, Wilkosz P, Tanbo TG, et al. 'Is unilateral oophorectomy associated with age at menopause? A population study (the HUNT2 Survey).' *Hum. Reprod.*, 2014, 29(4): 835–41. doi:10.1093/humrep/deu026
182 Hanley GE, Kwon JS, McAlpine JN, et al. 'Examining indicators of early menopause following opportunistic salpingectomy: A cohort study from British Columbia, Canada.' *Am. J. Obstet. Gynecol.*, 2020, 223(2): 221 e1–21 e11. doi:10.1016/j.ajog.2020.02.005
183 Reed SD, Newton KM, Thompson LB, et al. 'The incidence of repeat uterine surgery following myomectomy.' *J. Women's Health (Larchmt)*, 2006, 15(9): 1046–52. doi:10.1089/jwh.2006.15.1046
184 Bhave Chittawar P, Franik S, Pouwer AW, et al. 'Minimally invasive surgical techniques versus open myomectomy for uterine fibroids.' *Cochrane Database Syst. Rev.*, 2014, (10): CD004638. doi:10.1002/14651858.CD004638.pub3
185 Yuk JS, Kim M. 'Incidence rates of myomectomy-related mortality and venous thromboembolism in South Korea: A population-based study.' *Front. Med. (Lausanne)*, 2022, 9: 849660. doi:10.3389/fmed.2022.849660
186 Chrisman HB, Saker MB, Ryu RK, et al. 'The impact of uterine fibroid embolization on resumption of menses and ovarian function.' *J. Vasc. Interv. Radiol.*, 2000, 11(6): 699–703. doi:10.1016/s1051-0443(07)61627-3
187 Gupta JK, Sinha A, Lumsden MA, et al. 'Uterine artery embolization for symptomatic uterine fibroids.' *Cochrane Database Syst. Rev.*, 2014, (12): CD005073. doi:10.1002/14651858.CD005073.pub4
188 Mara M, Fucikova Z, Maskova J, et al. 'Uterine fibroid embolization versus myomectomy in women wishing to preserve fertility: Preliminary results of a randomized controlled trial.' *Eur. J. Obstet. Gynecol. Reprod. Biol.*, 2006, 126(2): 226–33. doi:10.1016/j.ejogrb.2005.10.008
189 Karlsen K, Hrobjartsson A, Korsholm M, et al. 'Fertility after uterine artery embolization of fibroids: A systematic review.' *Arch. Gynecol. Obstet.*, 2018, 297(1): 13–25. doi:10.1007/s00404-017-4566-7

List of resources

Endometriosis

The Endometriosis Foundation – a not-for-profit organisation dedicated to raising awareness and providing trusted and transparent information, education and support: https://www.theendometriosisfoundation.org/about-us

Endometriosis UK – a charity that provides information about endometriosis as well as hosting a free, confidential advice line: https://www.endometriosis-uk.org/

Adenomyosis

The Adeno Gang – a community created for those who suffer with adenomyosis to learn, educate and share knowledge about adenomyosis and menstrual health: https://www.theadenogang.com/

Fibroids

The White Dress Project – a US-based organisation raising global awareness of uterine fibroids: https://www.thewhitedressproject.org/

PCOS

Verity – a self-help group for women with PCOS, run by others with PCOS: http://www.verity-pcos.org.uk/

Premenstrual syndrome (PMS)/premenstrual dysphoric disorder (PMDD)

International Association for Premenstrual Disorders – provides support, information and resources on PMDD and premenstrual exacerbation: https://iapmd.org/

Support for women with premenstrual dysphoric disorder: https://www.mind.org.uk/information-support/types-of-mental-health-problems/premenstrual-dysphoric-disorder-pmdd/about-pmdd/

NHS advice: https://www.nhs.uk/conditions/pre-menstrual-syndrome/

Samaritans: www.samaritans.org

Premature menopause support

The Daisy Network – provides support to women who have been diagnosed with premature ovarian insufficiency (POI), and their partners and families: https://www.daisynetwork.org/

https://www.nhs.uk/conditions/early-menopause/

https://healthtalk.org/menopause/early-premature-menopause

https://www.nhsinform.scot/healthy-living/womens-health/later-years-around-50-years-and-over/menopause-and-post-menopause-health/early-and-premature-menopause

Dr Mandy Leonhardt and Dr Hannah Short (2022) *The Complete Guide to POI and Early Menopause*, Sheldon Press – this book is an incredibly thorough overview of POI and early menopause. It's a must-read for anyone experiencing it, or for clinicians treating women with this condition.

Menopause support

British Menopause Society – the specialist authority for menopause and post-reproductive health in the UK: https://thebms.org.uk/

The Menopause Charity – provides education on the perimenopause and the menopause: https://www.themenopausecharity.org/

Gynaecological cancers

The Eve Appeal – a charity raising funds for gynaecological cancer research and raising awareness of gynaecological health and symptoms relating to gynaecological cancers: https://eveappeal.org.uk/about-us/

Jo's Cervical Cancer Trust – a charity providing trustworthy information relating to cervical cancer prevention, diagnosis, treatment and care: https://www.jostrust.org.uk/

Ovarian Cancer Action – a charity raising awareness and funding research to improve treatment and survival rates of ovarian cancer: https://ovarian.org.uk/

Period advice for teenage girls

NHS advice: https://www.nhs.uk/conditions/periods/starting-periods/ and https://www.healthforteens.co.uk/growing-up/puberty/periods-just-the-facts/

Lil-Lets period advice: https://www.becomingateen.co.uk/advice-blog/periods

Advice on period products

The Period Lady – provides information and advice on all kinds of reusable period products: https://www.theperiod-lady.co.uk/

Contraception

The Lowdown – a very helpful website written by healthcare professionals with experience in prescribing contraception. It features reviews of all types and brands of contraception, written by users, so you can see what other people's experiences have been: www.thelowdown.com

Contraception Choices – a website developed by a team of doctors, nurses and researchers from University College London in collaboration with young women. Its aim is to help women decide which method of contraception might suit them best: https://www.contraceptionchoices.org/

Brook – a charity that supports people with their sexual health and wellbeing: https://www.brook.org.uk/topics/contraception/

Support for fertility issues

Fertility Friends – a forum community dedicated to infertility and fertility support: https://www.fertilityfriends.co.uk/

The Human Fertilisation & Embryology Authority – Impartial, accurate information about IVF, clinics and other fertility treatments from the UK government fertility regulator: https://www.hfea.gov.uk/

Surrogacy UK – a professional organisation that can help throughout your surrogacy journey: https://surrogacyuk.org/

Breast health

CoppaFeel! – a breast cancer awareness charity, with a brilliant website that contains information about breasts and how to check them: www.coppafeel.org

The NHS: https://www.nhs.uk/common-health-questions/lifestyle/how-should-i-check-my-breasts/

Counselling

NHS Talking Therapies – counselling and psychological therapies for mental health. You don't need a formal diagnosis, and you can either be referred by your GP or you can submit a self-referral via this website: https://www.nhs.uk/mental-health/talking-therapies-medicine-treatments/talking-therapies-and-counselling/nhs-talking-therapies/

Advice on diet/healthy eating

The Association of UK Dietitians (BDA): https://www.bda.uk.com/food-health/food-facts/nutrients-food-facts.html

Gynaecological health issues in the workplace

Adviser Plus – provides information for employers and HR departments on issues that may affect women in the workplace: https://adviserplus.com/insights/breaking-toboos-and-raising-awareness-of-womens-health-at-work/

Index